DO IT

LIFE LESSONS learned

The sections are all authentic and taken from my life – the good are for you, the ugly are stored away and the bad are brought to your attention, making them easier to avoid.

The insights are simply my mixes: to-do lists or not-to-do lists.

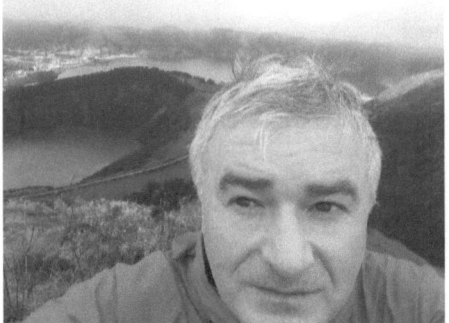

Name:	Franz Grubmüller,
Home:	Baden, Austria, EU
Born:	1961
Kids:	2 (adult)
Status:	Happy
Civil status:	Fixed partnership
E-mail:	franz.grubmueller@icloud.com

Table of Contents

DISCLAIMER

A broad range of diverse activities are listed in this book. Please use your common sense and consult a health care practitioner when undertaking anything which may be hazardous or even life threatening. Take proper medical supervision or consult a lawyer.

The author is not in any way responsible for any negative outcomes resulting directly or indirectly from information contained in this book.

FOREWORD

In my fifties I decided to write down my major movements, spiritual developments, insights into communication between individuals, managerial skills and my thoughts on mutual respect and drawing a red line through what is OK and what isn't. A moral compass. A kind of distilled content of my experiences when the margins, set by myself or by my environment, had to be extended. This was often connected with some sort of pain, when old habits had to be modified or deleted for new situations. How much has changed in these 50+ years! A lot, really.

Fortunately, I figured out that it would be easier for me and that I would have more success if I **changed myself,** just ONE person, rather than trying to change the other seven or eight billion people on earth or waiting for them to change.

Inspiring sayings:

An ounce of practice is better than tons of theory: Hariharananda, yoga teacher

You never plough a field by turning it over in your mind: Irish proverb

These sayings suggest that a "**DO IT**" attitude is what is effective, and things <u>not done</u> today might <u>never</u> get done!

If these insights don't wander from the brain (cool) to the heart (warm) they won't be forceful enough to initiate changes. I have a powerful vision in mind which could trigger the heart and thus empower you. The power of **positive emotions** makes this much easier than just using your intellect.

I see myself as slim, energetic, possessing many resources, happy and with a positive social field.

Therefore, I decided to treat my life as a unique possibility: <u>time should not be wasted by superficial talk, hate, jealousy or anger.</u>

<u>Practical matters:</u>

BOLD	**letters:**	**a positive attitude, to be encouraged**
<u>Underlined</u>	<u>letters:</u>	<u>to be avoided</u>
Italic	*letters*	quotes
<u>Italic</u>	***<u>letters:</u>***	***<u>internet links</u>***

The situations and insights in this book are from my life only. Summarizing everything in my book made the **DO's** and <u>DON'T's very evident</u> to me. When writing this book, I was able to figure out what life could offer. And it's not insignificant at all. No, it's tremendous!
The next challenge is how to practice all these good habits, and this question inevitably leads to chapter discipline!

Not all my wrong turns were significant enough to be mentioned here as DON'T's, and only the crucial issues and crossings have been highlighted.

Pictograms used

     Recommended book

     Link to a song

     Recommended movie

     EJECT: this sign means avoid this person, skip this behavior or quit!

     A not-inexpensive "medicine"

I have many good friends who have helped shape and challenge me; I really haven't achieved this all alone. My parents, my brothers and sister, my many relatives, my friends, my wives, my kids, my personal trainer, my physiotherapists, my orthopedist, my bosses, my yoga teachers, my colleagues, Dr. Eggetsberger and his family and a lot of good books and movies.

I know the advice and experiences given by my guests by heart. Their knowledge is a part of my life and is worth spreading and sharing for the greater good! A kind of expanded point of view.

Thanks also to Tim Ferris. His work, "*Tools of Titans*", pushed a button in me to pull my own strings and create this work. He did a GREAT JOB. It would be a pleasure for me to hammer a horseshoe for good luck at *Sepp's Place* together with him.

Pick out what's relevant to you and do your thing. I wish you the very best in accomplishing it!

I believe that we all are interconnected by some great mystery. This is a belief which underlines that our daily learnings are a shared achievement. This leads to shared lessons rather than ego lessons. Perhaps this is the counterpart to the current greater mainstream of egoism. I hope so.

Special thanks to Nicola Wilton for proofreading the manuscript.

https://language-boutique.de/wilton

I dedicate this book to my beloved mother, Antonia.

AS I BEGAN TO LOVE MYSELF

CHARLIE CHAPLIN on his 70th birthday

*As I began to love myself I found that anguish and emotional suffering are only warning signs that I was living against my own truth. Today, I know, this is **AUTHENTICITY**.*

*As I began to love myself I understood how much it can offend somebody as I try to force my desires on this person, even though I knew the time was not right and the person was not ready for it, and even though this person was me. Today I call it **RESPECT**.*

*As I began to love myself I stopped craving for a different life, and I could see that everything that surrounded me was inviting me to grow. Today I call it **MATURITY**.*

*As I began to love myself I understood that at any circumstance, I am in the right place at the right time, and everything happens at the exactly right moment, so I could be calm. Today I call it **SELF-CONFIDENCE**.*

*As I began to love myself I quit steeling my own time, and I stopped designing huge projects for the future. Today, I only do what brings me joy and happiness, things I love to do and that make my heart cheer, and I do them in my own way and in my own rhythm. Today I call it **SIMPLICITY**.*

*As I began to love myself I freed myself of anything that is no good for my health – food, people, things, situations, and everything that drew me down and away from myself. At first, I called this attitude a healthy egoism. Today I know it is **LOVE OF ONESELF**.*

*As I began to love myself I quit trying to always be right, and ever since I was wrong less of the time. Today I discovered that is **MODESTY**.*

*As I began to love myself I refused to go on living in the past and worry about the future. Now, I only live for the moment, where EVERYTHING is happening. Today I live each day, day by day, and I call it **FULFILLMENT**.*

*As I began to love myself I recognized that my mind can disturb me, and it can make me sick. But as I connected it to my heart, my mind became a valuable ally. Today I call this connection **WISDOM OF THE HEART**.*

*We no longer need to fear arguments, confrontations or any kind of problems with ourselves or others. Even stars collide, and out of their crashing new worlds are born. Today I know **THAT IS LIFE!***

These wonderful lines from a great comedian reflect a lot of my pursuits. Please forgive me for borrowing them.

They are great and inspiring, so let's begin!

LIFE PLAN

If you are hiking from A to B, you will most probably use a map to head into the right direction and you will consider the time, distance and the problems or opportunities between the start and the end.

In other words, you will have a plan.

You realize it is useful to have a plan for your education, your career, your family life and so on. Vacation plans are also included. We like to know that for short ranges we are strong and dedicated.

When it comes to a greater plan – for your life, for example, over 70 to 90 years, so that you see the sun on earth – this is another issue. I was the same ☹, or perhaps I still am. Suppressing our finiteness is common in our world.

Attending a funeral of a good friend or singing or listening to an emotional touching song, a song that rocks your soul and cleans away the dust and rust – this helped me confront my finiteness.

In der Mölltalleitn

In da Mölltålleitn, in da Sunnaseitn,
da san die Blüamalan noch amål so schöan.
Willst a Stäußle bindn, scheane Blüamlan finden,
muaßt in die Sunnaseitn einegeahn
Willst a Stäußle bindn, scheane Blüamlan finden,
muaßt in die Sunnaseitn einegeahn.

In da Mölltålleitn, in da Sunnaseitn,
da seind die Diandalan noch amål so schean.
willst a Diandle kriagn, willst di recht valiabn,
muaßt in die Sunnaseitn einegeahn.
willst a Diandle kriagn, willst di recht valiabn,
muaßt in die Sunnaseitn einegeahn.

In da Mölltålleitn in da Sunnaseitn,
do is dos Rostn noch amol so schen
Wånns mi aussestrågn auf an hölzarn Schrågn,
bleibts in da Sunnaseitn amoi stehn
Wånns mi aussestrågn auf an hölzarn Schrågn,
bleibts in da Sunnaseitn amoi stehn

Below is a brief translation from the Carinthian dialect into English (Carinthia is a beloved part of southern Austria).

On the sunny slope of Mölltal (the valley where the river Möll flows):

- The flowers are a little bit more beautiful. If you want to make a bouquet, find beautiful flowers, you must go to the sunny side
- The girls are much more beautiful. If you want a girl, to fall in love, you must go to the sunny side

- When I'm carried out, resting in a wooden coffin is more beautiful when you rest on the sunny side.

Life is not infinite. So, use this short time in a good way. Drafting a life plan could help you focus on the important milestones.

Input from a Viktor Frank Art Installation (Kloster Pernegg)

From	->	To
Who am I? (The past is over, it cannot be changed)		**What kind of person would I have been once?** (I can influence the future now to see the effect then)
Why me? (Victim)		**What is that challenge for?** (Participant who can adapt accordingly)
What do I need? (Me)		**What am I needed for?** (You)

What a person finally wants is not luck, but a reason to be lucky!
This is an introduction to reflect on the important content of your life plan.

The life plan, _**Living Forward**_, of Michael Hyatt and Daniel Harkavy gives a lot of practical insight into building the chapters right away.

Start at the end: **How would you like to be remembered when you are gone and passed away?   What is your life goal?**

How do I (Franz) want to be remembered?

God	Self-disciplined and spiritual; I see myself as part of the universe
Spouse	Funny, trustworthy, working on his assets
Kids	A good father, support in turbulent times
Parents	Family is my root
Partners	Genuine, smart, a top connector of people and systems, room for improvement
Friends	Helpful, open-minded

The five biggest regrets I want to avoid before death:

1. I wish I'd had the courage to live a life true to myself, not the life others expected of me.

2. I wish I hadn't worked so hard.

3. I wish I'd had the courage to express my feelings.

4. I wish I had stayed in touch with my friends.

5. I wish that I had let myself be happier.

Priorities: what matters most:

1. Health

2. Developing new systems, workflows, creativity

3. Savings

4. A strong family backgrounds

5. Spirituality

Action Plans: How can I get from here to where I want to be?

Account 1: **Self-Development**

Purpose Statement: Fully responsible for myself, great independence, great excellence

Envisioned Future: Be a top sparring partner for top management

Inspiring Quotes: Excellence in whatever I do; carpe diem

Current Reality: Finance manager for 30 years

Commitments: Job: Improve cost accounting
Utilize new digital tools like document reader

Privat: Improve video cutting skills (Wings Pro)
Produce fitness and chillout music tracks
Professional usage of GoPro camera
Write this book

Account 2: **Health**

Purpose Statement: Keep my body fit

Envisioned Future: Remain **lean** and strong, maintain good mobility and intact brain

Inspiring Quote: Move, dance, be born

Current Reality:
- Back pain   Do gymnastics
- 20 pounds too heavy   Skip dinner

Specific Commitments:
- **Stretching as a main goal**, shoulder exercises with TRX
  (= total resistance training), a form of suspension training that uses
  body weight exercises to develop strength, balance, flexibility and core
  stability.

- **Bike and hike** with film camera – capture the landscape
- Fitness club 3 times a week, sauna with cold water plunge
- <u>Reduce TV</u>
- **Regular meditation**
- **Healthy food and fasting as a cure**

Account 3: Wealth

Purpose Statement: Increase funds (see chapter CASH)
Inspiring Quote: Independence
Current Reality:

- House, flat
- Bank savings and insurances, cash = king

Specific Commitments:

- Fixed monthly saving in funds, i.e. spread risk

Account 4: Social

Purpose Statement: Be a trustful father, partner, friend
Envisioned Future: :-)
Inspiring Quote: A good friend
Current Reality: OK
Specific Commitments:

- Vacation with my kids
- Activities with Martina
- Trips with my friends
- Men's meeting once a month
- Doing sport with others

I review my plan every 6 months to control and, where necessary, adjust the direction.

This is MY mode of giving my life spin and drive and reducing irrelevances and distractions from the noise this modern life involves!

For someone else it may be simpler: to try and be happy every day. As people are different, so too are their modes and needs for improvement. I completely respect this.

CONSEQUENCE (Aurel Lackner)

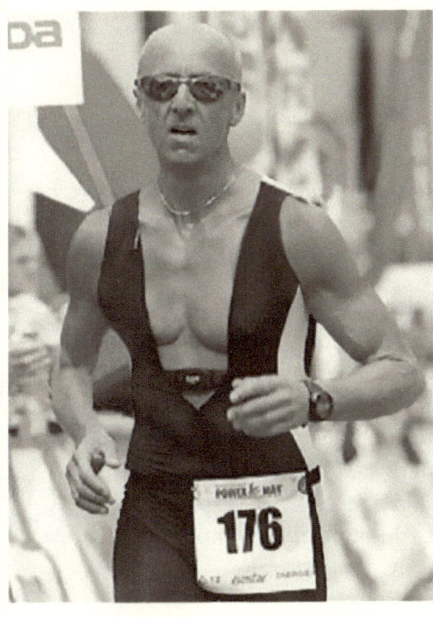

I failed my very first bike race – the www.velorun.at – which covered 53 miles and climbed an altitude of 1200 m. So, I asked Coach Aurel for professional help.

He convinced me to strengthen my total muscle tone from head to toe, so that the hands and feet don't "fall asleep" through intense exhaustion because the body can now support itself with a better muscle armor. This process was integrated with training to improve power and endurance, which are imperative for a faster recovery after tense climbing sessions.

It worked and I completed the distance successfully with a time of 3:40 h, or 14,5 miles/hour. Not bad for my 57 years.

Next step: under 3 hours ☺

Lesson learned: Set yourself high goals.

Let me introduce Aurel: www.fitness-sportconcept.at

Aurel did his apprenticeship in communications engineering at school and then founded his own electronic company providing parts for automobile businesses. He has always practiced sport at a high level, including judo, taekwondo and boxing. For him, this is a kind of basic exercise to train the will and strengthen the body.

He recently joined a foreign special military service for a year, drilling both body and mind to an ultimate level and extending his existing borders to a level yet unknown. Of 50 applicants, only two completed the "torture". And Aurel did it with bravura. Being tormented by trainers for the greater good is still not his fondest memory! His perception of the future was built on the most inconceivable pain that a body can endure.

His Mindset

- My Body   =   My capital
- To be healthy =   Attitude "produced" by consequent behavior
    - diversity in sport activities, even at night, because the days were dedicated to raising money
    - stretching is very important
    - healthy food and a low alcohol intake
    - because life runs at a high training level, every deviation disturbs the result
    - results driven means deviations in the long run are erased as far as possible
- No pain   =   No gain
- Decisions   =   clear commitment, no compromise

- Giving up is not an option and the meaning of the blues is unknown. Why? Simply because there is too much of a plan and constructive work to be done and this leaves no space for these ineffective options!

  Living life according to a strong life-long training plan leaves little room for these indulgences.

Lesson: **choose wisely** (and don't spoil yourself unnecessarily).

In 2006 he connected with the ski touring scene in Austria. Heavy with gear but filled with heart, he keeps up with the top members by maximizing will and effort and reducing total weight to a minimum. In practical terms this means summer clothes in an ass-cold winter! "If you wear clothes that are too warm, you'll lose time. It's that simple."

Clothing reduced to almost nothing sounds logical, but the consequence is constant exposure to freezing. People who narrow their mind like he does are more likely to be victims of frostbite – they are much tougher than the average person who would feel pain earlier and give in sooner. He is too much of a professional in this matter and once nearly lost one of his fingers. The physician said to him "Finger off". Aurel refused, rewarming his finger and enduring a truckload of incredible pain. A former famous Austrian skiing legend, Hans Enn, said once: "In ski races we are exposed 2 to 3 minutes to the ass cold winter weather. Considering your race duration of 3 to 4 hours, we are just wimps!"

Neuro Socks

These socks are designed to increase stability, energy levels and mobility. You can wear them with a business suit as well as during a workout. I bought a few pairs to help my weak Achilles heel. They also increase blood circulation which is helpful on cold days. Check them out in his online shop.

Advice for Increased Mobility in the Elderly
- Start early in youth
- If it's too late: **Start now**! Better late than never.
- **Conquer your own resistance**
- **Mix gymnastics and endurance**
- **Increase your muscles**
  - Muscles support joints and the musculoskeletal system
  - Muscles burn fat, which becomes more important as we age and the total metabolic system declines
- Add **variety** to your sporting activities with a minimum of 3 or, even better, 4 types of activities.
  - It is more interesting
  - It covers the body and mind in a more holistic way

What is the benefit of doing all of this? What do you gain for the pain?

HEALTH – and not only in youth. Health becomes more important the more we age. Aurel is a perfectly fit Dad and Granddad !

A variety of different sporting activities can be compared to playing the piano with its many different keys – variety gives another insight, another melody. And it is not only the body that will be thankful for the variety. The mind appreciates variety too because more braincells will have more duties to fulfill and may not rest, or rust.

My Choice

I once completed the Vienna City Marathon, but my two (for better balance ☺) aching Achilles heels means that running has become less of a good choice for me.

This setback could lead to either a victim's view of "Oh, poor me, the universe is against me, blah, blah blah…" or an actor's attitude of **"What's left?"**

Is the glass half empty of half full? That all depends on **what your truth is**. It depends on your beliefs.

Honestly, what was left for me was really a whole bunch of things:

- Biking with a racing bike
    - Together with social activities like "bike and wine" with Hillinger somewhere.
- Biking with a mountain bike to a limit of 170 heart strokes.
    - In a team this is a fun and chattery activity.
- Cross training activities while watching a motivating video (e.g. virtual active videos running on Matrix machines).
- Using the TRX Functional training facilities
- Sling training for muscle strength and stability
- Hiking in a group with a challenging route and a nice "after work" activity helps to open the minds and hearts of the group
- Sauna with a minimum of two peaks – then into the cool water pot for cooling down 5 to 8 minutes (brrrrr). Exposure to both temperatures helps decrease inflammation. Inflammation is the root of cancer, so preventing it is a good measure. And it is good for endurance too!
- Stretching the spine.
- Strengthening the lower body and upper body in the functional training zone.
- Swimming. This is one of the ultimate coordination trainings as it increases the neocortex links to rebuild and restructure. An antidote against Alzheimer's!
  I avoid drowning (or something quite close to it) at the very start to finally swim some hundred meters, which is a hammer for me ☺. It's possible! But a lot of training is necessary because the coordination is very unnatural at first. In the long run – much joy and a tremendous increase in both endurance and efficiency. For me, it's a master's degree, whew! And for you, a trainer is better than no trainer about the risk of drowning and being thankful for help in urgent situations.

CONSEQUENCE!

ONE

My life became complex.

I found myself with two types of computers – one for the office and one for my private life – and common standard apps and open source apps doing almost the same thing … <u>BUT …</u> not the same. I had different TV systems which were difficult to synchronize – let alone the increasing number of remote-control devices. My data was stored in both physical and digital formats. In digital format I had a variety of USB devices, copies of hard disk drives which were improved to a faster solid state drive, leading to an extra external hard disk drive for copies. And finally, I had two cloud storage solutions: the first was cheap, slow and limited in space, the second was a little bit quicker for mass storage with practically unlimited space and charges an annual fee.

The same was true elsewhere, with my many bank accounts, savings accounts and insurance contracts with different insurance companies and some overlaps. Controlling them all was a shit admin job. Also, I had a camera type A and a smaller camera type B, both good, but two different approaches …

I have socks in green, white, brown and black. Ah, and social media and different e-mail systems. A sport watch of type A and bike computer of type B, both connected to different apps.

When travelling I took my toiletries from the bathroom and on my return, I put them back in the bathroom. I picked up the technical equipment I needed for cameras, phones and smart watch loading devices before travelling and shoved it back in its place at home afterwards. Something was always lost in transit.

Then, finally:

- This led to a lot of burdensome interfaces
- Extra time was required for extra admin needs
- Sometimes I forgot things to take with me on my travels, or forgot to return them back at home
- I had no clue which data storage device was the most current

Whaaaaa! Wrong turn!

This bad situation was a result of <u>being possessed by things and processes </u>instead of the other way around.

I had to get back control:

- One computer system (hardware and software).
- One phone type
- A good GoPro for videos and a standard GoPro for photos; can be mounted simply on the arm; a low payload which adds more value for me then the better but clumsier camera.
- One app system for office packages – obviously the one that charges a fee was of a better quality.
- An NAS file server system, which is now THE no. 1 data storage place for me:
    - available via LAN, WAN, internet access and app

- o the digital archive can be opened to my relatives if I pass away
- o **a very simple file structure with less than 5 main files**; EVERYONE should grasp the meaning and content through sheer intuition
- o the most crucial files are copied once a week into my cloud (no. 1) automatically overnight
- o my partner has limited access to files which are handled as a team
- o reduced need for drop boxes
- o photos from cameras and phones are saved here too (one cloud solution less)

+ One savings account, insurances partly cancelled and switched to one company
+ Black socks for business, white socks for sport
+ One type of sport watch and bike computer with one app to control the total workout.
+ A travel bag in addition to my home things with:
  - o one toiletry bag
  - o one medical bag
  - o one battery charger with five outlets for the most necessary travel gadgets
+ Bike: copy of cash card, cash and most crucial medication; NO extra inflating tool to keep the weight down. In the event of a flat tire -> call Mama!
+ Delete unnecessary mobile apps to avoid confusion and time-consuming updates.

Time saved for the important things in life!

To boost productivity:

+ Start your day with a tight plan leaving empty spaces for "unforeseeable" tasks.
+ Follow this plan closely and concentrate.
+ Complex targets need calendar entries, otherwise they tend to be postponed due to procrastination. This doesn't only happen to big targets and sometimes life's ONE try is definitively better than two or more tries.
+ Divide huge tasks into smaller parts; if possible, delegate.
  Follow Julius Caesar: divide and conquer, smart man!
  Or follow Matsushita. He had to delegate because of his weak body and what he achieved was incredible.
  What one person can achieve in their lifetime is often incredible.
+ Recheck activities for yourself and your partners -> calendar entry!
+ Use Outlook wherever possible.
+ Combine and streamline parallel processes to the utmost, e.g.:
  - o Call friends or business partners **with preparation list**
  - o Take necessary breaks such as toilet breaks, making tea, small talk over coffee and by getting some fresh air and looking into the blue sky (we'll touch on this again later)
  - o Be prepared and ensure meeting attendees are also prepared, i.e. focus on this ONE issue
+ Learn OneNote to structure your tasks: this tool uses ALL MS-Office file types including Outlook e-mails which you can easily structure in the register (on top) and in chapters (separate "pages").
+ Use the favorites in your browser, open multiple windows at the same time.
+ Your standard source should not be the sub/sub/sub file, but on top or in your favorites list. If you do not oblige it, your Pareto ratio will switch to 20/80 too, but 20 being productive and

the 80 unproductive. Open your standard programs ONCE a day when you start. For me it looks like this:

Job	Outlook	Excel	ERP	Browser	ONE			Explorer 2x (for copy)
Private	Outlook for	Browser			ONE	Word	Video	Explorer 2x (for copy)
	Gmx, iCloud	Server Music, Notes	Translater	Google				

Probably the most important task in these modern days of social media (a kind of Samsara) is to **concentrate on ONE task at a time!** Every day. ONE task at a time with full concentration. In the long run this is a lot of time gained for improved productivity. For your life!

A good teacher at a university explained to the auditorium for higher level accounting where the splitting of companies into an ownership and an operating unit was the topic:
"I know I'll request a lot. And you think when following me on the whiteboard you understand. I tell you: it is not that way! This was my experience as a student. It's heavy.
When you are at home and try to rethink the processes by yourself you'll find out that parts of the reconciliation chain you couldn't grasp, connect paragraph A tax law with paragraph Z and explain this with commercial law paragraph 123. So, please, for your own sake: **LEARN consequently and to the core. Learn ONCE.**"

You could delve into some lessons on productivity (and learn some German too) here:

 Steigern Sie Ihre Produktivität Jetzt! by Hartmut Sieck

The book includes many practical helpers for daily life.

Finally, ONE > TWO in terms of simplicity (yep, mathematically this is nonsense, I know. Dear maths teacher, please forgive me).

Simplify, Simplify!   5 -> 4 -> 3 -> 2 -> **1**

DIGITAL OFFICE

"Everything has its place, and everything has one place" is a basic principle of kaizen.

Outlook

Try to concentrate on one task means that **either you read and analyze, or you write**.
Mixing both tasks is often a strong challenge to efficiency and is reactive rather than proactive.

Psychologically, it's better for the mind to "run in front" rather than being pushed from behind. It's your choice.

In your e-mail "options" you can switch off the buttons that notify you of the arrival of new e-mails (sound, envelope sign etc.).

This frees your productive energy. **Do the same with your mobile phone and iPad.**

Rules for the in-box:

- **Open e-mails once,** don't waste time with multiple visits to ONE issue .
- **I leave e-mails in the in-box when not completely resolved**; this could take time if it is complex – then it stays in pending (on my table).
- **Reduce the content in your in-box asap,** it isn't a storage place and therefore it should be reduced for better transparency.
- **Rename the subject** if the original wording is not specific enough.

- **Have courage – press delete if it's really garbage.**

- Avoid a superficial treatment of answers – this inevitably leads to the reopening of tasks. The check wasn't paid! Have patience and endurance!

- **Answer** it according to what it is:
  - simply file it if it was just fyi, daily reports, adverts, etc.
  - **an in-depth analysis and answer** for difficult tasks which need thinking, group discussions; further steps to be taken to solve the issue
  - **an e-mail could simply be applied to a calendar entry or shifted to the task list** so that further working steps and corresponding e-mails can be matched

Rules for the outbox:

- **Leave it in the outbox as a pending issue if no satisfying answer was received;** in the course of life I've learned not to treat things as done if they have just begun.

- People are different. "Remind" them of open tasks; depending on whether they are disciples or bosses, match their individual behavior pattern accordingly or use the company's general pattern.
  This could be as follows:
  - a formal call

- an informal call to start with then switch the topic to the task itself. State your mode of working and note that an unresolved issue will remain open if not completely resolved. This will convey your thinking not only now, but also in the future. The patterns will slowly adapt ☺
- an e-mail reminder
- an e-mail reminder querying whether everything was clear or if anything was misunderstood. This is politer (and humble)

- **Reminders are essential!** People tend to forget, especially when they become older. Me too!

- Attach a file to an e-mail using the **"attach file"** button. All recently used files will be shown. This is far easier then clicking through a complex folder hierarchy.

- **By using copy and paste a content will then be copied, and a new item can be created:**
  - in Outlook
  - as a calendar entry
  - as a new contact

  A great short cut combination!

File structure:

In-box

Outbox

And then a ten-folder (maximum) structure without sub-folders to keep track of your records. I sort them by starting with "0", followed by "1", "2" ...

Again, an absence of planning requires a tenfold payment in the construction! **It is amazing how much can be foreseen with professional planning.**

Saving time:

- If a task is very complicated, the in-box or outbox is not the correct tool. Rather create one or more comprehensive tasks covering the complex issue in depth. In the to-do list, the heading could be adapted to reflect the issue.
- Flags could simply be colored to separate them for different issues, e.g.
  - Job 1: red
  - Job 2: blue
  - ...
- You can apply flags simultaneously by using the CTRL or the shift key to select several e-mails at once.
- If someone addresses you using the cc, give him a call requesting direct addressing.

- My activities and decisions are executed in the following preferred way:
  - Modeling: **Discuss the issue personally** and structure the problem. In the modeling phase of new steps, flexibility is needed.

- o **Decision:** This should be **in a written format,** because this communicates a clear commitment.

- Avoid addressing three or more people in the address line if only one is doing the job! The rest should simply be informed in a cc.

- Use the **SEARCH function** when you don't know where an e-mail has been filed.

- Use "Quick Steps" (standard procedures for messages) as often as possible:
  - o first personalize your Quick Step with the NEW functions you require, and DELETE the stuff that is not appropriate for you, e.g. task, calendar appointment and drag and drop to your favorite folder
  - o then use it when you analyze e-mails and structure your answers

- Use a **clear subject.** This reduces reading time on the partner's side.

- If e-mails are sent around in a ping-pong game, the content tends to change. This requires an adapted subject.

- If possible, only discuss **one issue per one e -mail,** not more. This simplifies things.

- I prefer, as an example, "**kind regards**" to "KR" as this is more respectful towards the partner. I like to be treated in this way and so I should begin correctly – the karma or echo principle!

- **I explain my moves so that my counterpart gets my intention**. This needs more time in the beginning, but it attracts your partners to you instead of just "using" them as an answering machine. I recall times when I explained new things to my kids when they were growing up. I like to be treated in the same way – again, the karma or echo principle ☺

- Before pressing SEND: read and check the content to see if it is fluently written and understandable, if the content is logical, if the correct commands are used and if the wording is polite.

  My mother once told me: Never write a letter in anger!

Read more of these insights in this most valuable blog:

10-ways-to-work-more-efficiently-in-outlook/

Other Hints

I use the data path in footers for easier location of the file on the server. This is the correct procedure for internal documents but may not be suitable for external documents.

If useful info relating to a partner arrives on your table, place this **partner information in the address book in the notes field immediately:** e.g. Doctor Schiwago, open Tue 8.00 – 12:00. Do this as soon as you receive the information, not later, because the pile of information will grow together with the distractions.

If my **PIN** for a bank account is, for e.g., 4578, I use a backup note, **simply adding, for e.g., 3 at the** end. This comes to 4581 (4578 + 3). If applied to my other PINs it's a kind of track for me only – I must only recall "3" and "+."

File name conventions and storage places:

Naming convention should be strict.

190528_Project Calculation 2018 which makes it easy to find and sort. The updated file days later will then be named 190601_Project Calculation 2018. And sorting from top to bottom is easy.

Old and obsolete files in the working folder are simply shifted to the sub directory "OLD" so they aren't lost but are removed from daily sight.

Again, **ONE file only!**   Version 2 and 3 -> Folder OLD

Link function:

Your file structure should be similar to this:

Folder	Sub-folder	Sub-sub-folder	Files
House			
	Invoices		1,2,3,4,5
	Costs		6
	Projects		7,8,9,10,11,
Kids			
	Money		12,13,14
	Vacation		15
	School		16,17
Documents			
	School		18,19
	Job		20
		Contracts	21,22,23
		Application	25
	Offical		30,31,32,33,34

This provides a good clear picture. You don't like to change this structure because it is yours!

But it's difficult to **find the most important files in one place only.**

This puzzle isn't difficult to solve:

Folder	Subfolder	Sub Sub Folder	Files
House			
	Invoices		1,2,3,4,5
	Costs		**6**
	Projects		7,8,9,10,**11**,
Kids			
	Money		12,13,14
	Vacation		**15**
	School		16,17
Documents			
	School		18,19
	Job		20
		Contracts	21,22,23
		Application	25
	offical		30,31,32,**33,34**
Basics			**Link 6,11,15,33,34**

You need to link the highlighted files into the MAIN folder "Basics" using the Windows symbolic link function! Both advantages are covered: **One storage place and one "pick-up" place.**

OneNote (Software) and OneDrive (Storage)

These MS cloud solutions have the following advantages:

- **Access from everywhere**
- **Front-end facilities are supported: desktop, iPad, iPhone**
- Backup provided by MS
- **Multi-user access** (read only or read and write) if access has been granted by the owner
- **ALL MS File types** can be used (e.g. Word, Excel, PowerPoint, Outlook, …) as well as **audio, video and text boxes**
- Very clear structure in **chapters** (upper level) and **register** (lower level)

A top tool worth delving into!

OneNote and OneDrive may also be reached by internal and external partners.

Examples:

1. Private: Shared vacation plan (Papa, kids, travel agent)
2. Job: Shared job description of colleague retiring soon (him, me, colleagues)

KAIZEN

Kaizen is a Japanese philosophy behind an Eastern technique for simplifying life. It's a process of **continuous improvement** indicating change (KAI) to become good (ZEN).

In short, it is the "Toyota Way" which was developed after WW2.

Explanation of "5S":

1. SORT: When in doubt, move it out

2. SET in ORDER: A place for everything and everything in its place

3. SHINE: Clean and inspect **or** inspect through cleaning

4. STANDARDIZE: Make up the rules, follow and enforce them

5. SUSTAIN: Make it a part of your daily work and it will become a habit

PDCA Cycle

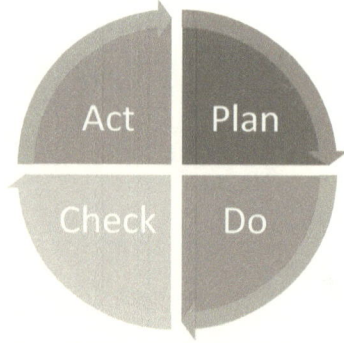

Continuous improvement:

Following these guidelines leads to a reduction in exceptions, a reduction in disruptive interfaces and, ultimately, preparation for digital processing.

A colleague of mine once said: "Franz, if you have a shit process transferred into a digital model, you'll get a shit digital process. First, the process must be cleaned!"

REDUCE

Now: Distraction, commerce and food everywhere –> filling the head, heart, belly, house or flat with a lot of things, thoughts and noise. Music everywhere. And the world is so small and easily reached by plane. Mass tourism? NO, billions of individual tourists!

Then: In childhood I didn't miss the important things like clothes (they were often second-hand), food (it was simple and enough), love and care from parents. We didn't have many things, so I looked forward to getting a pair of skis to share with my brother – and it worked. I saved money for a year to buy my first calculator in technical school. We often made our vacations in mind only – following our fingers on the map. Tourists in those times were called strangers. Buying a ticket from Europe to the USA cost a fortune, leaving us dollar-less when we arrived. My very first travels abroad were on a low budget and with much hope and joy. I even saw the two World Trade Center towers, both still standing in NYC.

I don't want to turn back the wheel of time; change is the only constant thing in life. It is more to reflect on the core of important issues in life, because I was once happy with a smaller pocket. It is to limit the number of things and influences in your daily life, because, for e.g., 5 issues are easier to control than 10 or more. It is about eliminating distractors and seeing what is important.

A famous yoga teacher named Paramahamsa Prajnananda was once invited as a guest somewhere in the West. He did a world trip with a small trolley and was invited to store his clothes in the host's cabinet. He saw the cabinet brimming with clothes. Comparing both he asked his host: "Do you really need so many clothes?

My father was born in 1931 and was transferred from Carinthia to his home village near me. He came along with a puppet-sized suitcase! **He didn't need more.**

 "We may idealize freedom, but when it comes to our habits, we are completely enslaved." ***The key for fortunate balance in modern life is simplicity.***
— Sogyal Rinpoche, *The Tibetan Book of Living and Dying*.
Reading and learning from this man is always inspiring.

"And as long you haven't died, rise and be, you are just a dull guest on the dark earth." Johann Wolfgang Goethe. Sorry for the bumpy translation, but he was THE German poet.

"A clear 'no' is better than a forced 'yes'." My mother.

"Oh, how void, oh how elusive is man's life ..." The first line of a song taught to us in school by our music teacher, Mr. Schlögl.

Do I really need so many clothes? Are my gathered habits any good for living my life? Is this a free life I'm living or an attached life; attached to daily distractions like TV, surfing on the Internet, reading newspapers, social networking, relaxing with a good glass (or more) of wine, buying things by simply pushing a button … and the logistics (and its waste) have started. Am I willing to let go of things, thoughts, good or bad experiences, fears …?

What is the positive impact of reducing?   **Simplicity**

Is there a fear of losing the distractors which are preventing me from hearing the silence within me?

Habits could be obstacles on the way

In my childhood, I learned that proper behavior was sometimes rewarded with a gift. These patterns have intensified to become a part of my character. This means that they were deepened and are no longer superficial. Patterns are repeated, like in Groundhog Day, leaving Phil in a time loop that is very hard to escape. He had to turn the wheel 20 or 30 times to find the way out.

In short: think -> do -> do again -> habit -> character – and there we have the mess or the wonder.

For some lessons I learned in former times it is déjà vu. But this is not necessarily always positive. It's even worse: they become worthless and even incriminating.
Examples:

1. Food is the reward for a tough day, consequently more food is a bigger reward
2. Relaxing alcohol = the way out of stress
3. TV as a distractor to relax PLUS chips

Feel free to compile YOUR List, you have the grace of privacy.
I must stand tall and bright and cannot hide anything in the name of authenticity, uff! ☺

Too much of the above has left me heavy and dizzy and, in the end, has reduced my power levels, either in my job or in private activities with friends and family. These are not good habits, that is for sure. But there is always a place for short-minded thinking

Way out?

AIM HIGH, this gives you a long-term goal to accomplish. The next step is to make the goal manageable – divide it into chapters and follow the plan in a bullheaded manner. The consequences are crucial. Frankly speaking, **work your ass off** and put everything into the pot! If you failed once at attempting a goal set high, when one day you have success, the honor is great. This is a real boost! I've done it and it sounds and feels good.

Example:

-   2017 I tried a marathon bike race over 50 miles with an altitude difference of 1100 m and failed
-   2018 I succeeded with a time of 3 hours and 40 minutes because of my intense indoor preparation
-   Next year I'll be back under 3 hours by reducing my weight by **20 pounds** – and hopefully within the main group of bikers

REDUCING is the key to perceiving the important things in life.

PRESENTATION

Preparation

A good presentation needs a lot of thinking, feeling and preparation in advance to match the needs of the audience (and yourself). A one-hour presentation requires 20 hours of preparation.

Negative impressions remain far more easily in the mind than positive impressions. So, mind your step!

What's the title?

Which auditorium?

What is my intention? I must know what the outcome will be, the result of the speech.

> This is important only for me

> This mentally streamlines me

> This intention comes into force by my doing

General

Personal impact is

- ➢ 55%   non-verbal signals
- ➢ 38%   voice
- ➢ 7%   content

Steady eye contact

Present the ideas with confidence

Open posture

Mindset: ☺

Arms above the waistline deliver a proactive and positive signal

Loud and firm voice

	"I" to be mentioned rarely
Show and explain slide A	Don't show slide A while discussing slide B People will be confused
Talk in pictures	Avoid spreadsheets with 1,000 numbers
Most important content: repeat 4x!	Or it's forgotten

Begin

Open question — Avoid closed (yes/no) questions

e.g. What's the picture of our balance sheet?

Which beginning to choose? Dramaturgy! Either:

- Play some music – and stop abruptly!
- Throw a bag of money onto the table and shout: "Let's burn cash!"
- Remain silent for a minute – a signal for concentration in the audience

Wait for late listeners, positive	<u>Don't punish them</u>
"I welcome you"	<u>Not, "I'd like to welcome you"</u>
	<u>Avoid we should, would and could</u>

Content

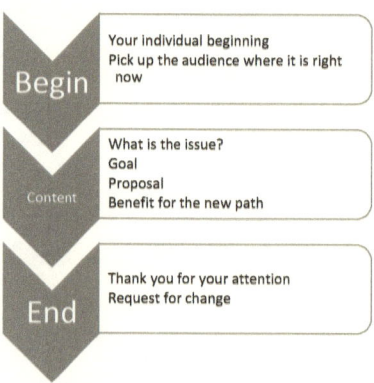

Begin
Your individual beginning
Pick up the audience where it is right now

Content
What is the issue?
Goal
Proposal
Benefit for the new path

End
Thank you for your attention
Request for change

Info block for 1-3 minutes

1 picture per info block

Most important issues should be reinforced with pictures

Animation if it's helpful and not distracting

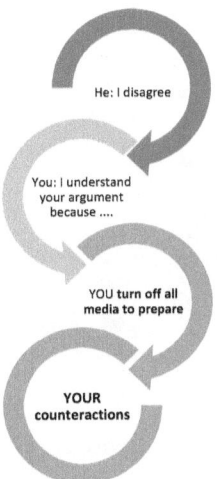

He: I disagree

You: I understand your argument because ....

YOU **turn off all media to prepare**

YOUR counteractions

Do not fight against opposition.

It requires courage to say: "At the moment I've no argument for you. I'll have to analyze this and will revert back to you."

MANAGEMENT

Task

Communication

Whatever the problems we must deal with are, the **basic requirement is GOOD COMMUNICATION** with your partners, and even your opposition. Without communication you cannot start analyzing tasks. Communication can be compared to developing the same language. Good communication pays off on good **and** bad days.

Communication:

- **Regular formal and informal talks** to get a feeling for where people are and to understand their motivations.

- **Regular information about the status of the situation** – colleagues should be treated as equals and not as poorly informed workers.

  The latter approach is very common in hierarchical companies. Knowledge equals power and power and knowledge is always concentrated on TOP and usually not distributed as this would erode the power level. This is very common in the EU. Information flows upstream.

  I believe that a corporation becomes stronger and can grow more through distributing knowledge and intelligence to its peripheries. This is more common in US companies.

- **List of team members, their duties, the interfaces and the tools.**

- Again, only **one**, because two or three means extra work in translating, interfacing and so on:

    - language
    - place of data storage
    - collaboration platform
    - environment:
        - test: to be used for test purposes
        - production: the go – live environment
    - project e-mail folders in which tasks are separated instead of being fed to all the members in their e-mail boxes

    - agreed form of memo to document progress which has the advantage of being split into:
        - Done
        - Open

From this, you can easily see the progress from the very beginning, you can scan through GREY areas and scroll forward to open issues. Open issues are always, so to speak, "on top."

But you always have the past as a track record, i.e. what has already been done.
It's very useful to have this information in three years' time for when your boss asks you:

"What happened in year 4?" In this case, you will have the information available in the most recent memo. Yep!

Day 1	Day 10	Day 20	Day 40
Issue 1	Issue 1 (grey = done)	Issue 1 (done)	Issue 1 (done)
Issue 2	Issue 2	Issue 2 a (done)	Issue 2 a (done)
	Issue 3	Issue 2 b	Issue 2 b (done)
		Issue 3	Issue 3
			Issue 4

"Our life is frittered away by detail. Simplify, simplify." Henri David Thoreau

- Have the guts and talk to the opposition.
  Listen to what he has to say and reflect on your own decisions. Emotion is human, consider this.

    - **Treat the opposition with respect, but have courage**

    - Don't try to simply smile and ignore the conflict. Sometimes a fight is necessary!

- **Note and reflect on deviations from the plan.** Use a "compass". When heading west you'll not reach north. If you don't see the deviation, you'll not be able to navigate or steer back into the right direction. Deviations could also be "mistakes", but this is life.

  Reinhold Messner, the first man to summit the 14 highest mountains in the world, had more abandoned projects because of bad situations than successful ones. This wise attitude most probably saved his life more than once.

- **Sometimes a beer** achieves more than tons of workshops and protocols.

- **Listen more than you talk**, because you will learn from your partner instead of filling someone else with your own knowledge. This requires humility, which may be difficult for the western guy who prefers to talk rather than listen. Listening indicates respect for and attention towards your partners.

- **Increase your standing:**
  - call your partner by his name; "Hello Frank"   =   personal
  - a firm handshake shows confidence   =   you are strong
  - look them in the eye   =   confidence, no fear
  - repeat what they said in your own words   =   interest and reflection

- Simple, **genuine interest in your partner** is 90% of a good "sale." It is astonishing how much people are only interested in themselves, circling around their own center, closed to new inspiration – we live in an EGOISTIC world!

 How to Win Friends & Influence People, Dale Carnegie
Written in 1936 and still valid!

Don't forget: Our world is full of egoists. A real **interest in other people** will give you an advantage. This goes against the mainstream and it will most probably result in a smile on the other person's face.

"You can make more friends in two months by becoming interested in other people than in two years by trying to get people interested in you." Dale Carnegie

- <u>Don't intend</u>

  Instead turn on marathon mode:
  - vision
  - evidence collection
  - proof
  - concept draft
    - WRITTEN
    - benefit is or will be
    - team and responsibilities
    - environment for testing or reality

- steps …
- GO or NOGO
  - concept improved or approved
  - kick off
  - doing
  - error assessment -> error correction
  - new trial 1
  - improved picture but not satisfactory?
  - next trial

Do not forget Edison: "One percent inspiration, **99 percent perspiration.**"
Vision as a source of power is necessary when things go wrong.

- Have great **respect for your colleagues.**
  "Always be kind, for everyone is fighting a hard battle." Plato

- Give everyone **his share of responsibility**, don't treat anyone as just a stupid helper.
  In the long run, people will identify more with their tasks. Let your people earn their medals
  and they will take the blows if things go wrong.

- **Criticizing the bad things and praise the good things** means you see their contribution.
  Errors should not be "ploughed under." Learn and improve the next time round.
  Allowing errors to "burn" without giving them attention or using the fire extinguisher is
  never a good idea. You are weak and blind, without ambition, like a flag lost to the spinning
  wind – no power!

  *"A life spent making mistakes is not only more honorable but more useful than a life doing
  nothing."* George Bernard Shaw

  No mistakes = nothing done   ->   **TRY**

- Treat people as they are – different. There is no standard recipe for everyone. This means
  that a lot of talking is needed to understand and improve the situation.

- Instead of simply giving orders - **make contracts with your partner!**

  In the long run this behavior is more successful than simply giving orders.
  I must remind myself of this quite often.

- Look for the **benefits to your colleagues**! Try to see it with their eyes: **What's their future
  benefit?**

- Change your perspective. Adapt to the role of an external adviser if you are too absorbed in
  daily problems. See the problem from a distance. Reflect from a distance.
  A day off before making tough decisions could be helpful.

  "It is a common experience that a problem difficult at night is resolved in the morning after

the committee of sleep has worked on it." John Steinbeck

- **Lead through query:**
  The one asking the challenging questions is leading someone to the answer.

- Keep yourself inspired. This gives a better vision and better endurance.

  "Twenty years from now you will be more disappointed by the things you didn't do than the ones you did. So, throw off the bowlines. Sail away from the safe harbor. Catch the trade winds in your sails. Explore. Dream. Discover." Mark Twain

- <u>Rambling speakers within earshot?</u>
  - o make contact
  - o adapt to their rhythm
  - o pick out one word matching your proposed context
  - o grasp the lead and follow your proposal, denying them by looking in another direction
  - o well done!

- People who are attracted by perfectionism usually dislike new things in which they are not confident. Perfectionism (usually the known environment) ≠ risk (usually the new environment).

Recently I gave some of my new insights space to develop and thus needed to abandon old habits. Everything has enriched my life. But I must confess that it is not only Bruce Willis, but also old habits, that die hard!

Winners and losers

"Winners have good Ideas – losers have good excuses." Unknown

"Negative people have a problem for every solution." Albert Einstein

Surround yourself with winners and avoid naysayers, troublemakers and blockheads. And if that is not possible, change their attitudes to solution-creators. Changing their attitudes is a long process and, according to my experience, involves blood sweat and tears. Much easier is charisma. But I have still not found a shop that sells this. So, I took the long way around. But feel free to take the short cut. And I would be delighted to hear about your expertise later – I'll listen.

"If you know your enemy and you know yourself, you need not fear the result of a hundred battles." Sun Tzu

Dalai Lama
"If you think you are too small to make a difference, try sleeping with a mosquito!"

The Dalai Lama and Laurens van den Muyzenberg have produced a wise book on management:

The Leader's Way: The Art of Making the Right Decisions in Our Careers, Our Companies, and the World at Large

Extract:

- Develop your view: In order to lead, you must understand the reasons for your actions. As the Dalai Lama says, "The nature of our motivation determines the character of our work." **What is the intention behind a decision?** The decision should be for the benefit of the whole company.

- Establish the right conduct: In order to ensure your best intentions are consistently applied to your business practices, **develop a system of regular progress reports** and evaluations.

- Train your mind: You lose your calmness when you <u>are angry.</u> An absence of calmness in your mind means an absence of steady thinking and reflection and <u>no clear decision</u>. **Simple meditation techniques such as deep breathing, muscle relaxation and controlled emotions can help even the busiest leaders keep composed.**

      ->   Alpha – Type

"A man is but the product of his thoughts. What he thinks he becomes."
Mahatma Gandhi

- **Focus on happiness:** **A happy company is a successful company**. You are more invested in success when you care about where it comes from.
And don't forget: **It is impossible to be angry and happy at the same time!**
If you choose happiness you will be boosted more than if you go on grumbling about this and that and what has been done against you.

  "Always laugh when you can. It is cheap medicine." Lord Byron

- **Become interconnected:** It is the leader's job to manage and reinvigorate impulses among colleagues. Remember that interconnectedness does not only mean relationships within the company, but also relationships with clients, customers, the financial community and even competitors.

- **Stay positive:** Appreciate how rare and full of potential your situation is in this world – take joy in it and use it to your best advantage. **Every problem has a solution** and having the right attitude from the beginning may help you find it.

  "I am an optimist. It doesn't seem too much use in being anything else." Winston Churchill

I have summarized how an enterprise resource planning (ERP) migration project could work out positively on LinkedIn:

Critical success-factors in an ERP-migration-project Franz Grubmüller

- **fast Close** in the old ERP System = shorten the gap
- **flat hierarchy** within the (small) project Team = fast & motivating
- **crystal clear workload definition** for each member = no excuses
- communication: long-range **planned meetings** & reports as well as **ad hoc meetings** / telephone conferences if " a fire occurs somewhere"
- use the setup of the **new IT company = learn their language** = faster & more structured & delivers respect
- **2 to 3 test migrations** needed = improve & learn prior to Go Live
- Close contact to all included colleges = **training & motivation**
- **allow emotions but don't forget a beer :-)**

Reinhold_Messner

 Reinhold Messner is a famous European mountain climber and the first man to summit the 14 highest mountains in the world – all above 8,000 m. He also trains managers. The essence of this is can be found in his book:
Berge versetzen: Risiko-Management in Perfektion

(translated as Move Mountains: Risk Management in Perfection, available in German only, no Kindle version)

He talks a lot about his motivation for doing these great and dangerous things. He describes it as a spinning flywheel which straightens him into an "upright" position after having failed at something difficult. He "feeds" this motivation by developing highly ambitious visions.

Extracts from this visionary book:

- *Mountains to move are inside your mind.*

- *People who perform their tasks wholeheartedly and with joy and enthusiasm will have success. Vitality releases energy.*

- *If you don't try new experiences, you remain static. If you undertake second-hand experiences, you only consume.*

- *I'm telling my truth, although I know this makes me unpopular.*

- *First comes the idea, then follows the method of realization and finally the risk management.*

- *Dogmatic paradigms and entrenched habits must be avoided.*

- *Calculate to include possible errors. An intolerant error strategy is cruel.*

- *Having the guts to take risks provokes new discoveries.*

- *Great respect for a big goal challenges the best within my personality.*

- *If a leader sets inspiration free in each team member, this will be matched with success and invincibility.*

- *Motivation cannot really be bought.*

- *Avoid free riders. They know how to get the most credit out of the smallest possible commitment.*

In my understanding, Messner says that:

1. first a person must lead himself in a good and inspired way
2. the rest will then follow

Matsushita Leadership, John P. Kotter

 Matsushita was the founder of Japan's General Electric. What has been achieved by this man is incredible – the greatest increase in sales in the 20th Century in the lifetime of the founder!

His initial situation:

- born into poverty
- lack of basic education
- lack of money
- lack of a structured business plan
- poor health
- not handsome
- stopped by the Great Depression

Would you believe in such a man? Would you give him money for his ideas?

As seen from my standpoint, I doubt it!

When reading the story of his life I often had tears in my eyes. I very quickly stopped complaining about my situation because it was zero in comparison!

What was the motor within in this man?

His beliefs!

A BIG VISION! And the intention to achieve it!

His life lessons were:

- **take full responsibility for everything in your life**
- **always see the very best of people**
- **hardships in life can be survived**
    - **take risks and explore new paths**
    - **hardship shapes character**
- **Be open-minded and humble**
- **Go from passive consumer thinking ⇢ active producer thinking (from reactive -> to proactive)**
- **I always have a free choice in my life**
- **I will bring value to the people for their benefit and will do them good**
- **challenge the status quo to aspire to higher things**

The Concert, Radu Mihaileanu

This film gives you an idea of how inspiration for a great idea could change people's minds! People go from the lowest to the highest mountains of self-development and don't let the naysayers prevail.

The story in short (without divulging too much):
A dismissed orchestra group had a stroke of luck with the chance to perform a violin concert far away from Moscow, somewhere in Paris. The processes involved in coordinating people, gear and money to perform a famous violin concert are funny and inspiring, while at the same time very melancholic. Music is a carrier for people's visions, who are sometimes on the brink of abandoning this "crazy" idea; pain when people's borders are challenged. In the long run it is a great JOY!

Problems and worries?

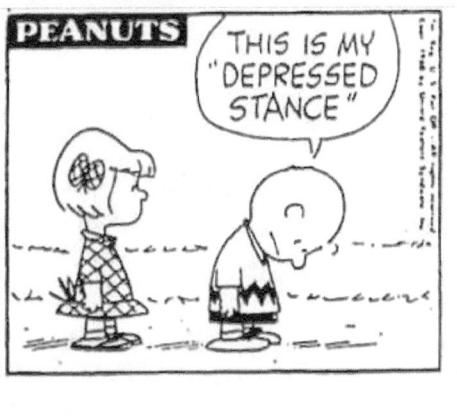
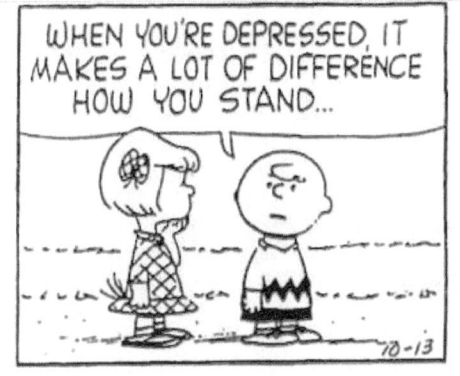
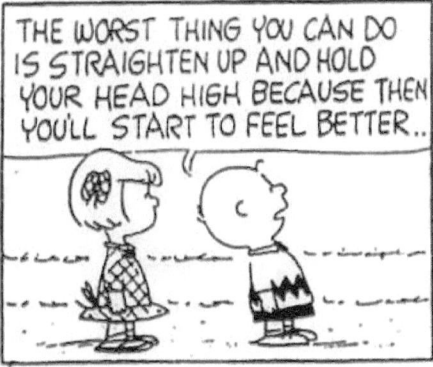
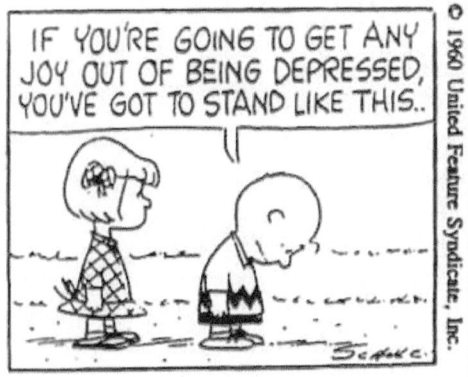

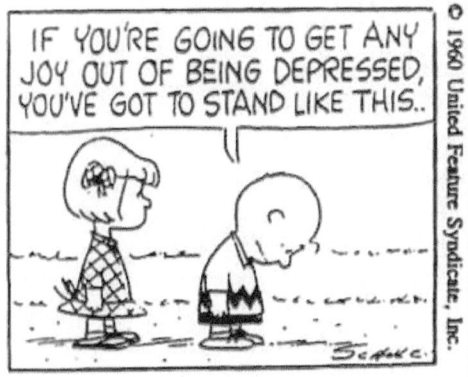 *How to Stop Worrying and Start Living, Dale Carnegie*

Dale Carnegie's experiences in 1940 as an adult teacher offering practical advice to his pupils are still valid in our modern times.
An evergreen!

Have dreams and live them

LIFE IS MY TEACHER
(Herwig Fohrafellner)

Reflections on Mauritius, January 5th, 2019

"Life is my teacher." A coconut salesman here in Mauritius told us this yesterday because he also spoke a little German. When Carima, my wife, and I asked him who taught him this, he just said in German: Life is my teacher.

That's why I want to write down something here that life has taught me so far. The eternal question of life: Why are we here? What are we doing on this planet? What am I doing in this world? Over the years of observing what is valid here on earth and possibly even in the rest of the universe, I have noticed the following:

-   constant return
-   nothing is wasted

Nature creates a rhythm of constant return, night and day, the seasons, birth and death. In this constant hustle and bustle and changing of things, however, there is one constant: Even the smallest of things are used and utilized regardless of where they are located. Each leaf that falls from the tree is reintegrated into the eternal cycle of being and not being, where the respective being is represented only in its present appearance. It is used in all cases and by being a leaf it had meaning and value. Would it not, therefore, be illogical if we human beings did not also have meaning and value in our being? In my opinion, this logic lies in the exploitation of our shell by millions of microorganisms, thereby ensuring their survival. The real value and meaning of every life, however, lies in the exploitation of the leftover energy, the soul, of every living being.

Of course, you can discuss whether this soul exists. My answer is a clear "yes" to this question. Life is my teacher. The only real death I have ever seen was my father, Stefan. I experienced him in the prime of his vitality and incredible strength. But I also stood by his deathbed. His facial expression and his face alone had changed to such an extent that I believe that something had left his body. My mother ran away when she looked into her mother's dead and lifeless eyes as she didn't recognize them.

Scientists have reportedly tried to measure the dying in absolute closed conditions, before and after death. A weight loss of 21 grams has been noted. The soul's measurements are of no consequence, but what is certain is that it exists. Since it certainly exists, the question is, what happens to it and what is it needed for? Remember the two basic principles:

-   constant return
-   nothing is wasted

The same must be valid again. Science now assumes that in about 100 trillion earth years, the entire universe will burn out and after this there will be no more stars and no more suns. At present, an infinite amount of energy is being burned in a billion suns throughout the universe. How many of these are in our galaxy alone? More than 300 billion? And in 100 trillion years they are all supposed to have burned out. What happens then? Is that really the end? I'm saying a clear no.

The only process in the whole universe where energy remains is when life dies. It would be ludicrous if it was precisely this process that made no sense. It is precisely this process that is the very meaning of our lives and our existence. The energy is recycled just like everything else. Energy cannot be destroyed, it can only be transformed. Now what is it converted and recycled into?

For those who believe, even God still has a place here, because is there really a God? If a God exists, then it exists only if there is also a universe. What does an almighty God do when there is no more? What, then, would be God's real purpose? In its divine dimensions, this is relatively soon, a palpable 100 trillion earth years. That could be the equivalent of a heartbeat for us. Yes, but what should God do and what is God's task when everything is consumed and burned out and there is no energy left, only a freezing cold zero degrees Kelvin in space.

Or isn't it? My energy is still there, as well as that of my wife and children, those of my future descendants and those of my ancestors. The energy of the first human being is even still there. The energy of the recently-deceased fly next to me and the thousands of billions of deceased creatures that populated and populate this earth is still there. And wait again, even the falling leaf that I held in my hands this morning. Didn't that possess energy, too? If all this energy is still present, but the universe is over, wouldn't it be logical to reuse that energy, just as everything is reused? To create the whole universe again? Where does this take us? Exactly – to the next Big Bang. That is, mine, yours and any other energy ever generated in the universe serves only to enable all of us to live on through

- constant return
- nothing is wasted.

But since it is obvious that the energy generated here on earth is not enough to create a new Big Bang, we know that life must prevail throughout the universe, that in the next Big Bang, death leads to new life. We die to live. Now we could take another step and figure out how many earths it would take to provide the energy needed for another Big Bang in 100 trillion earth years. Let us just assume that we know how much energy is released by dying life each year and we assume that the earth will generate about 1.7 billion years of energy, then we just need to get the energy of the Big Bang through the energy of here on earth. The energy generated divides and we have several busy earths in our universe. But this calculation is incidental, because if the theory is correct then we know:

1. Our lives have meaning
2. Life goes on and on

For there is constant return and nothing is wasted.

It is, of course, very difficult to turn this doctrine into a religious message. Had I told my strictly faithful Catholic grandmother at the time: "Grandma, you were once used to create a new Big Bang," she would have wondered if I had had a bang and she would have excommunicated me on the spot. But even here, the divine doctrine, which is published in almost all world religions, still has a place. God needs quite a lot of heavily enriched energy to produce an as-good-as-good and loud Big Bang as possible. Good energy certainly has a higher energy potential than bad energy. That is why all the good things we do in our lives can serve to bring our energy potential to a higher, stronger level. So, we are more valuable to God but above all more valuable to space and the next universe. That's why all we must be is GOOD. We really should all try. Strive to do good and to love, because that's the ultimate form of GOOD.

Franz:

What does this philosopher do for daily living?

Herwig was keen on building tree houses. So he learned it professionally by getting an education in construction. At that time, fathers made the decisions! My father too. Herwig had to join a technical school learning to construct tractors and ploughs. I did the same as the son of a farmer. From a tree down to the soil! Thanks to this life lottery we got to know each other and ever since then we have remained friends.

After his professional career adventures in dangerous places like Iraq during the Iran-Iraq war, he founded a company called _Penthouse Construction_, building bigger "Tree Houses" ☺. More expensive, but far nicer and much more exquiste.

He once quarreled with his fitness club and subsequently quit. The private fitness room didn't offer the right challenges. So what came next? He opened his own fitness club, _Penthouse Sports._ This place is highly recommended for vicitms willing to lose some weight (and perhaps some more money as well).

A funny and prosperous man, who took his blows and follows his vision steadily.

HEALTH

People around me convinced me in more intake of fresh energy, which is practically speaking more of warm food and warm water because my body wouldn't have to heat up cool energy intake. With rising age, the inner battery declined, and I conceded in eating **warm food**.

My Morning Routine

- I open the window to get some fresh air into my lungs – a deep inhalation.
- I drink a small cup of Vitalogic.
- In the bathroom I give my thyroids a small massage.
- Before my morning toilette, I give myself an old-fashioned shave with a sharp blade.
  A promise: You'll concentrate completely, otherwise it could end up in a bloody mess. When I wasn't that skilled my face was often butchered, and plasters were required ☺
- The shower finishes with a cold plunge. After this I am fully awake!
- Warm breakfast (as described later in the text) and lots of coffee.
  When I was a boy of five or six, I had the chance to see my Grandpa drink coffee. He didn't use a cup – oh no, he used a big bowl containing roughly 1-2 liters. The little boy entered a new world: the adult's world.
- A short meditation starting with breathing and inward concentration. At the end I visualize the successes which will follow in the day.
- On the way to the office I massage the thyroid and/or the PCE muscle contraction combined with breathing exercises.

Tony Robbins' Morning Priming Routine

"Whenever you want to make a change or improve something, the first place you want to prove it is in your mental, emotional state. If you do something from a pissed off state, from an exhausted state, from a frustrated state, from a weak state, it won't matter what you do. The thoughts are weak when you're in a weak place. The actions are weak."

Priming, then, is intended to get you into an energized, positive state that will carry you through the day.

"If you don't have 10 f—ing minutes for your life, you don't have a life."

Tony Robbins' Morning Routine

Food and Exercise

My favorites scientists to follow by reading or listening to their podcasts when it comes to food and fasting are *Dr. Rhonda Patrick, Dr. Frank Madeo* and *Dr. Valter LONGO*. They all share an interest in preventing illness, pursuing longevity and providing optimal, lifelong health.

Please understand that our health system is guided by the pharmaceutical industry. And then some (very smart) people said that during fasting you could skip or reduce your pharmaceutical supplements. It's difficult to believe. I saw an old black and white movie from Lake Baikal where lots of diseases (e.g. joint problems, problems with the lungs, high blood pressure, etc.) were cured simply by:

Eating nothing and drinking only water for two or three weeks. Incredible! Old wisdom forgotten.

Every major religion has a fasting period during the year. These ancient societies knew why. Nowadays, we have too much useless information in the air and have forgotten the good wisdom. The old wisdom must be refreshed.

<u>**Prevent inflammation which is the precursor of tumors and cancer:**</u>

- Eat vegetables as much as possible, especially kale, broccoli and sprouts, and use turmeric.

  Consider that gorillas have much more muscles and power than man – on a diet of vegetables only. So much for the suggestion that mankind needs animal proteins! Our genetic similarity to the gorilla is nearly 100%.

  In my agricultural school we were taught that about 3 kg of flour is needed to produce 1 kg of meat (pork of course, it's the cheapest). The ratio is even higher for cattle and does not consider water consumption which increases the carbon footprint even more. This gives us another reason to eat more vegetables and grains.

- Use a sauna regularly as it works against inflammation and enhances endurance. Repeat 2x as a minimum and take a rest between the cycles. As bolster I often use a small furled towel.

- Take a bath in (very) cold water since it clears and enlightens the mind, reduces inflammation and increases the fat burning rate and strengthens the immune system. But please consult your physician to check whether the cold is good for your heart. Don't do anything stupid.

- Studies have shown that a cool down after exercise could counteract endurance. A better sequence is:

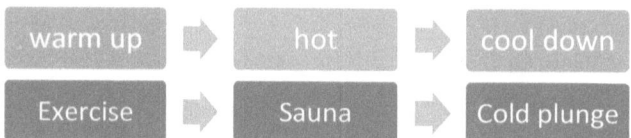

… and not the other way around

- Salmon twice a week is recommended and boosts heart health. If I do not eat fish, I supplement with omega-3 fish oil.
- Cancer loves simple meals like sugar. I reduce my sugar consumption as much as possible, which is good for the body shape too ☺ A problem for me is that alcohol contains carbohydrates chemically like sugar. This means that alcohol must be limited too. Uff!
- If sugar, then dark chocolate!
- I also add whey to my diet to help the ankles and joints. Vitamin D levels should increase since this improves metabolic efficiency. Recently, my physician complained about my vitamin D levels being far too high – he'd never seen this before. I had to reduce the dosage :-)

Others:

- Most water intake should be before 3 p.m. to reduce toilet breaks which disturb sleep.
- Rather read a book at night than watch TV because the TV light doesn't make you sleepy. Books do! Absorb the blue of the heaven during the day.

- I do my physical training by biking or cross-training at least twice a week. If I'm in training for a competition (provided my Achilles heels are fine) then this is far more intense.

  My resting heart rate is below 60 when in intensive training. The same happens when I'm fasting. If the total amount of heartbeats per life is limited (which it is!), then training is good for a long life!

- I do my stretching every Sunday in a workout group.

- I take a garlic and lemon mixture once a day in the morning against calcification – sobering, brrrrr. To make this, cut seven organic lemons into pieces and take out the pips because they will taste bitter. Cut a handful of garlic into pieces. Put everything together with 1 liter of water into a blender. The pulp should then boil for a minimum of 2 minutes on the stove. Filter after boiling and you have your liquid cure ready to be filled into a clear bottle. Every morning drink one small glass of garlic and lemon mixture to reduce calcification. I do 2 cycles a year.

Acid – Alkaline Food Chart

To make life a little more complicated I'll now stress the importance of the acid or alkali content of food and drink. Obviously, one should have a higher alkali intake than acidic. The problem is simple: many delicious foods and drinks are acidic or even highly acidic ☹ What a pity!

Let's start with a shortcut to give a simpler overview of the next task in your labyrinthine struggle:

Acidic	Neutral	Alkali
Soya beans	Beans	
Beer, Cola, Soft drinks, Vodka	Water, Apple juice	Ginger tea
Bread	Cereals (no sugar)	
Hard Cheese, Cheese	Butter, Milk	Fruits
Beef		Vegetables
Other Meat; Fish		
Walnuts, Peanuts	Almond, Flaxseed, Macadamia	Hazelnuts, Pumpkin Seed
Sugar	Honey	

The ultimate acid-alkali food and drink chart

You can delve in here for more details.

Spermidine

The older an organism, the less Spermidine it produces. Spermidine was originally found in semen and is good for:

- a strong heart and longevity
- increasing brain memory and reducing the risk of dementia
- activating autophagy

You get it from eating (this is my way):

Mushrooms, chickpeas, peas, apples, grapes, ripe cheese, soya beans, grain bread (organic), potatoes, nuts, vegetable sprouts (wheat bran, pine nuts).

Or as supplement (this is not my way).

Glycaemic Index

The glycemic index (GI) is a ranking of foods containing carbohydrates and their effect on blood glucose levels. So, you'll find no meat in this chapter.
A high index indicates a fast increase in glucose and a fast decline, i.e. the saturation period is short.
A low index indicates a slow increase in glucose and a longer saturation period.
Even the cooking process can impact the GI of a food. Over-cooked spaghetti has a higher GI than "al dente". Ah, **spaghetti al dente!**

high	medium	low
Glucose, White bread	Brown rice	Peanuts; Lentils
Baked potatoes, Fries	Honey	Bean sprouts, Chickpeas
Popcorn, Chips	Oatmeal	Grapefruit
Beer	Macaroni	Spaghetti al dente
Watermelon	Organic bread	Carrots, Vegetables in general
		Oranges, Bananas

https://www.curejoy.com/content/high-glycemic-index-fruits-and-vegetables/

This means that a TV evening with beer and chips is an accelerator for increased consumption, generating hunger while filling the stomach. Beer simply shouldn't be part of a daily diet and should be consumed very rarely.

My Breakfast

General advice: Cook your vegetables so they are close to raw.
A warm up in the morning will do the rest of the cooking.

Breakfast 1

1. Red onions and shallots   1a. Kale, broccoli into a pot with water, 10 minutes cooking
2. Some carrots
3. A little bit of ginger
4. Avocados, walnut, flaxseed, sesame seed
5. Kale and broccoli and a little bit of red wine
6. Tomatoes, bananas, whey, raisins, mushrooms, wheat bran, chickpeas, beetroot, dates

7. Pepper, paprika, turmeric, lemon (not too much and not too little), parsley, cranberry, coriander

Variation

- Coconut milk or yoghurt
- Spinach and/or mangold, asparagus, fennel, artichoke or kelp
- Rice or spaghetti or potatoes
- Salmon or chicken or tuna from a can

My wife isn't too happy when she meets an odor of fish in the morning.
But, no pain (for her) means no gain (for me)! To some extent, she has finally conceded. She also complains about the turmeric stains in the kitchen – what a shame, this short-sighted point of view.

I started with a regular-sized pan, but I now prepare breakfast for some days in a row!

After letting it cool:

1. A fresh plate is on my breakfast table
2. The next two days' worth goes into the refrigerator
3. The rest goes into the freezer

For aesthetic reasons I separate my food into three pots – almost beautiful in my eyes, of course ☺

1. Vegetables
2. Meat or fish
3. Rice or spaghetti

The cooking time is 30+ minutes in total, including preparation time. According to my wife (I'm not so fussy), the kitchen afterwards is a disaster.

Looking at the huge amount of ingredients, it's obvious you can create many variations.

Breakfast 2   (preparation in the evening)

1. Cereal (no refined sugar)
2. Apple sauce and water (1:1)
3. Walnut, flaxseed, sesame seed
4. Whey, raisins, wheat bran
5. Chickpeas, figs, dates

Variation on top of the bowl   (in the morning)

- Fresh bananas, grapes
- Peas, apples, oranges, melon
- Blueberries on top

Cinnamon and cacao (bitter, without sugar) at the end as a topping.

Breakfast is the most important meal for me. My body is hungry after 16 hours without food and the new day starts with energy intake.

And for a carbon dioxide balance: buy local and seasonal products.

Whenever you enjoy a good meal, do it wholeheartedly and with great joy, and celebrate it as if it's your last. Life is too short to crucify yourself for enjoying it.

If needed (to adjust for yesterday's effect) **add a day of fasting or skip one or two meals, also with a full heart and with enjoyment**.

There is just a small decision needed to spin the wheel.

No Food = Fasting

No food means only water or tea without sugar. Please note: Drink less mineral water and plainer tap water since mineral water can't wash out old garbage that easily. The longer you plan to fast, the more mineral water you can drink because it supplies mineral salts.

Also, no water out of plastic bottles since this will weaken your bones.

Some of the effects of fasting:

- ➤ Apoptosis: damaged cells are self-destructed
- ➤ Autophagia: damaged cells are eliminated and used for energy (eaten)
- ➤ Stem cells increase: these are the "repair mechanism" in our body
- ➤ Ketosis: when damaged cells and carbohydrates aren't available, the body turns to fat cells for its energy

Thus, fasting resets our immune system, reduces inflammation, strengthens age-damaged cells (increase in lifespan) and, as a bonus, fat is burned!

It looks like our body is better prepared for longer periods without food than with food. Starvation periods were quite normal in the development of our species. We had to survive these periods with less carbohydrates by adopting a protection mode. It looks like this protocol is stored in our genes as well as in the genes of animals who most likely had hunger periods too. Ancient mechanisms direct the body into protection mode.

When the body switches to ketosis mode (1–2 days after the beginning of the fast) the mind becomes clearer. This is an effect of ketosis (fat-burning) which provides a steadier supply of energy than that from carbohydrates.

Cancer cells don't have this old protection mode. Therefore, they are severely inflected (reduced) during fasting. This means that fasting is a complementary action against cancer. Even chemotherapy is more easily tolerated with 2 or 3 days of fasting prior to the chemotherapy. I know that if I am ever diagnosed with cancer, I'll prepare myself by fasting to reduce the torture of chemotherapy!

Modern times with tables and fridges filled to the brim make survival more of a challenge – diabetes, obesity, high blood pressure and heart diseases are increasingly prevalent. Mankind isn't wired for abundance. It's a strange modern world.

Some methods described below vary in the time required.

1. Time restricted eating or, in old-fashioned words, cancelling dinner

This refers to a **non-feeding window longer than 12 hours,** or, even better, 16 hours. In practice this means no food after 5 p.m. until breakfast the next morning for me. Don't forget that this means no food, no coffee and no alcohol, just water or sugar-free tea. This starts the daily repair-mechanism of autophagy. Over time, the pounds will drop. This method allows you to easily keep your weight steady.

The Italian types amongst us will probably die without dinner, Mama Mia, so they will skip breakfast or lunch instead.

If a social evening is on the radar, I'll skip the next lunch.

Consuming a lot of water is a key factor for reducing the appetite and supporting the cleaning process.

2. Fasting for 2-3 days

This is an experience that resets our immune system by releasing old trash to rejuvenate. To withstand the process, it is very important that **even more water** is consumed for washing out the old cells. A minimum of 3 liters per day is necessary, and 4 or even up to 6 liters is better. This is because the cleaning process can be painful, and the body is supported by large amounts of water to help with the washing out. Most of the water intake should be before 3 p.m. to ensure that sleep is not disrupted.

When fasting, I suffer from headaches and painful sciatica. Movement, in the form of brisk walking for an hour or more per day, is critical. This stimulates blood circulation and prevents a build-up of negative effects. **Saunas** can help to transport "waste" out of the body. A mandatory **liver wrap** should be applied once a day. This supports the liver in its job of detoxification and starts the ketosis process for energy supply.

You could simply integrate a 2-3-day course as a "no food" period into your timetable without being bound to starting with fasting and then afterwards starting with refeeding.

3.) Fasting > 3 days

When fasting for 4-7 days (or more), an increase in all the positive effects is much higher but the process itself is trickier:

- The bowel must be cleared, which is normally done through an **enema**. This is not rocket science, but it should be done with care. Your bowel should be emptied every second day to completely clean out the old waste products which are most likely to send poisons back into the body and result in headaches.

  If you need extra support in getting rid of everything in the bowel I highly recommend **colon**

hydrotherapy which is a "full-service" enema to remove waste products.
The effect:

- fungi, viruses, waste products hindering digestion and poisons are washed out
- the absorption of vitamins will improve, and general strength levels will rise

Not a very fancy method, I must admit. It's taken me some time, but I finally concede that it's worth it. The effect on me is that I'm not at all hungry after six days of fasting and so I decided to extend my fast for another two days. Colleagues of mine did 10 days of fasting and had to inject some force to start themselves eating again! It seems that the body goes into a completely different mode (ketosis) and by feeding itself it gains confidence in itself – a wonder!

- Refeeding after the fasting period should start slowly, because after one week of water you won't easily be able to digest fat products and only very light products are good for your stomach.

- Generally, it is advisable that these longer durations are done in a specialized camp with supervision and not on your own.

Lesson learned:

Fasting is a trigger for better health and longer life.

In greater terms, this leads to healthier people needing less medication and perhaps medical treatment – an enormous effect.

How that would crash into our GDP model which is based on growth rates instead of reduction or, at the very least, stagnation! What happens if people start forgoing food for periods of time in their lives – what if this becomes mainstream? What happens if vegetable consumption increases and meat consumption decreases? How does this affect all the parties involved in this process?

The impact would be great, but a better world would be waiting. More vegetables would lead to reduced energy consumption (remember the minimum 1:3 ratio of flour to meat), which means more food for everyone. Starvation around the globe would decrease, consumption in total would decrease slightly and mankind would be forced to adapt for survival.

I did several courses at the Kloster Pernegg guided by Evelyne who did a great job both in the course and in the "after sales" time! Evelyne did some treatments in Sri Lanka which is a most inspiring place for fasting.

https://www.klosterpernegg.at/begleiter/schneider-evelyne/

You can put it as simply as my girlfriend when she teases me sometimes about my searching for better ways to live: "Eat less than you need. Reduce drinking (alcohol)" ☺

Alkali Bath

If the feet smell there is more out of balance than the bad smell indicates. A "sour" climate results in a bad body odor and is the base condition for nail and foot fungal infections. If these "products" are detected, you know that there are too many toxic substances in the body.

Since the feet are the most distant parts of the body, they should be given some extra help with this bath procedure. These special bath salts have a pH value of 8,5 which helps to eliminate toxic material via the skin. The soles have multiple reflexology points responsible for detoxification. This bath supports your fasting side effects which could result in body pain because of the slow process of washing out the sour climate. Subconsciously, one may be reminded of the time in the mother's womb which provided the same alkali climate for detoxifying our body via the skin.

I do this once a week for a minimum of one hour as a precaution. Music or a book can give you company. Brushing the whole body regularly helps get rid of the old cells.

Effect:

- Detoxification sucks out the bad sour climate of our body
- In so doing, it eliminates the basis for fungi (which likes acidic areas)
- This results in a much better body odor, including the feet
- This works against heel spurs
- Reduces skin calluses
- A wonderful relaxation hour ☺

Jentschura My Base Bath Salts, Amazon

Be patient with the timeline of your detox. The problem didn't arrive overnight. Take your time and include this pleasant procedure in your routine.

If you don't possess a bathtub or you'd like to focus on your feet only, use a footbath and enjoy the time! Your feet will say "thank you very much" either way.

By the way, these feet carry us over our whole life – they deserve some support.

Go barefoot as often as possible – it is good for the feet and your health in general.

In order to help your body rid itself of toxic materials, the direction of brushing the body is important for maximizing the positive stimuli.

Brushing of the body in direction of precipitation

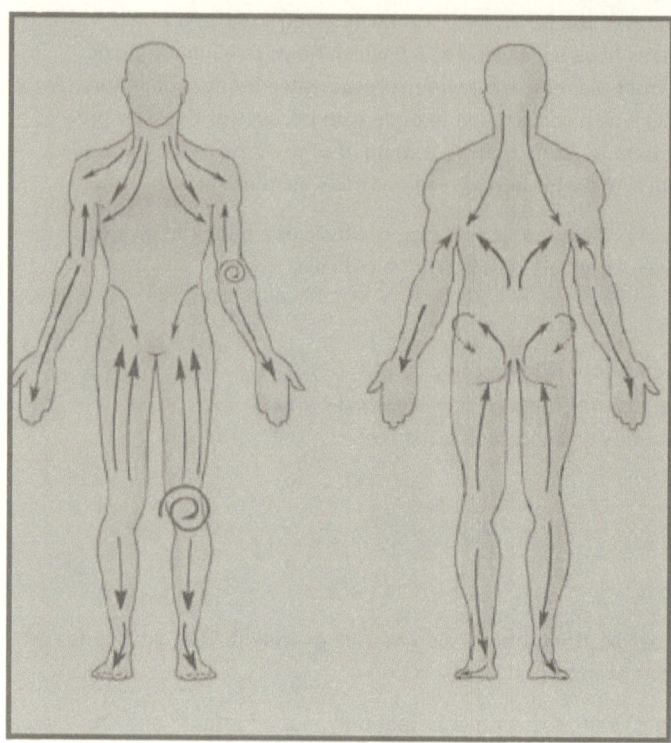

My personal experiences:

My heel spur would need classical surgery resulting in six weeks in plaster and a long time for recovery. I tried to get rid of the fungus in different ways, including pills and tinctures, all to no avail. The reason is simple. The sour climate in my body (stress) kept inviting the fungus in, again and again. The answer is another kind of climate change.

Body odor improves relatively quickly, and the rest requires patient and constant treatment.

Enjoy a nice bath

Uña de Gato / Cat's Claw

I attended a shamanic training in Austria where I got to know Don Pedro from Peru. This guy was talking about a very special training down in the jungle while his friends were playing around with girls. He was strictly committed to learn in the woods. As far as I understood, his efforts paid off (at least in the long run) since the knowledge of this rural man is impressive. There are so many natural pharmaceutical remedies found in the jungle that can help in natural cures that it was difficult for me, as a newcomer, to follow.

He was hesitant in giving his core medicine freely to the audience since his colleagues have complained of institutions which are well known in Latin America stealing this information. He stood tall and opened his knowledge to the audience.

Liana, or cat's claw, is a plant growing only in the jungles of Peru and is used to cure pulmonary inflammations, and general inflammation problems in general. This drug is one of the main medicines the jungle has to offer to the rural people.

An Austrian citizen staying in Peru lost his comrade to cancer. He contacted rural people in their primitive huts full of smoke from ovens without chimneys. He wondered why there were not more chronic diseases caused by the thick smoke. The people drank lots of tea made from cat's claw.

Years later I attended a Spanish training course in Quito, Ecuador, and found this drug again at a market. My language teacher Anabel regularly sends me more of this liana. Thanks a lot, Anabel.

Since 2005 I have used liana as a tea while at the office.

I almost never catch a cold!

Vitalogic

 A friend of mine works as a coach in the biking scene in Austria. His advice to boost endurance, shorten recovery time and increase strength by avoiding drugs is a tailored mix of amino acids.

Look at their website here: *Vitalogic*

Its function is simple: A blood test reveals peaks or deficiencies in essential amino acids. Here you'll see my sample list:

Franz Grubmüller 17.04.1961 Blut vom: 25.12.2018

Essentielle Aminosäuren	Ergebnis (µmol/l)		
* Arginin	13	[x--------]	8
Histidin	40	[--x------]	22
Isoleucin	60	[----x----]	28
Leucin	96	[---x-----]	59
* Lysin	66	[x--------]	63
Methionin	15	[--x------]	10
* Phenylalanin	45	[-x-------]	37
* Threonin	75	[-x-------]	54
* Tryptophan	24	[x--------]	24
Valin	159	[---x-----]	105
Essentielle Aminosäure Derivate			
Neuroendokriner Metabolismus			
* Glycin	213	[x-------]	207
Serin	140	[--x------]	79
* Taurin	149	[-x-------]	124
* Tyrosin	45	[-x-------]	36
Ammoniak/Energiemetabolismus			
- Asparagin	34	[x ---------]	42
Asparaginsäure	92	[----x-----]	26
* Citrullin	17	[x-------]	16
* Glutaminsäure	128	[--x------]	97
* Glutamin	232	[-x-------]	209
* Ornithin	69	[-x-------]	50

Poor levels of:

<u>Bad mood:</u>   phenylaniline, tryptophan and tyrosine

<u>Tired:</u>   threonine, glutamine and ornithine

The cost per month is approximately 100 USD, so it's not a cheap medicine.

From your results, an appropriate mixture of essential amino acids will then be prepared for you and this powder should be taken twice a day.

My personal perception is:

More energy, better mood.

Sleep

I sleep on an average 7 to 8 hours per day during the week, and a little more than 8 hours over the weekend. Using the weekend to catch up on loss of sleep does not eliminate the bad influences on your health. It's much better to maintain a constant sleeping time in order let your body rest and recover during the night.

Please do a self-test and check if your weekend sleep without an alarm clock is significantly longer than during the week. If yes, you need to increase your sleep time during the week!

Good preparation for the night:

- The greatest part of liquid consumption should be finished before 4 p.m. – toilet breaks will be reduced.
- <u>Avoid mobile phones</u> and computers in the evening – blue light indicates daylight.
- <u>Avoid TV</u> – it is not good for relaxation.
- **Go for a walk.**
- **Read a book.**
- **A brief meditation for 9 minutes before going asleep** will provide a tremendous boost for a good and relaxing sleep. This investment will pay off soon since recovery is better.

PCE Yoga (Jenny Fox)

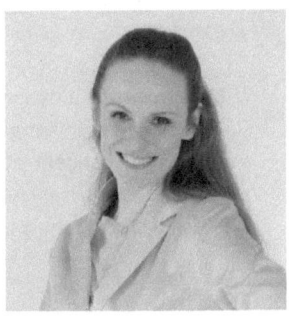

Jenny Fox is a very good trainer of PCE yoga thanks to her dancing experience. She explains the theory behind this yoga.

The PCE yoga exercises deal with the increase of the flow of life energy. This involves rune exercises (yoga), energy exercises (PC muscle training) and corresponding breathing exercises. The goal is to optimize the energy levels in both body and mind by steady training. This improves performance in everyday life, has a balancing and harmonizing effect and shows a significant improvement in stress resistance in different life situations.

The life energy originates in the pelvic floor muscles, the pubococcygeus (PC) muscle. The PC muscle is a cross-striped muscle that runs between the pubis and coccyx. When used properly, this muscle produces large amounts of energy which is transported through the spinal cord into the brain and into every single cell of the body. Regular exercising transforms this muscle into an energy generator.

By tensing the PC muscle, women stimulate the uterus and men the prostrate, leading to a release of hormones and endorphins which can cause mental elation, for example during sex. The activation of energy from this inner power center **increases mental activity** and **stimulates power.**

By using the rune exercises (the PCE yoga exercises) **body tensions are dissolved**. They kickstart the natural, ever-present life energy. The functions of the glands are also activated and thus help us towards inner harmony. The PC muscle is the source of life and thus sexuality and sexual energy. By using PC muscle training, you can lift your overall energy level and cognitive abilities!

Scientific explanation (Dr. Gerhard Eggetsberger):
 www.pep-live.com

Franz:

When one feels stressed and the shoulder and neck regions are tensed, then it's time for a relaxation activity. In my world, this is **every day**! It helps one **let loose** and this is my challenge. If I'm not relaxed, then the flow of energy through my body and mind is blocked or at least hindered. This means that life could be experienced at less than 100%, behind a thin fog and with half the output. The energy won't flow then, and the battery is low.

Detach …

These exercises combine:

1. **Rune exercises** most probably invented by Celts. All exercises are done **when standing** erect. This, again, is ancient wisdom and to some extent lost knowledge and has been reactivated by Dr Eggetsberger.

    and

2. **PC muscle contractions**. The main function is to stop urine flow. If this works correctly, it can benefit both men and women. The advantage of this should not be underestimated because

it means that we could save a lot on adult nappies in our old age!

Another advantage is **a positive igniting of the brain,** like sex fuelling the brain, which sounds archaic but is nevertheless essential for reproduction. Brain and sex work together for the greater good.

Why is this such a dynamo for energy?
Simply because this organ is responsible for the survival of mankind and therefore has this much power concentrated in it. This muscle fires energy through the spine into the brain which chooses wisely where the best prospects for offspring are ☺
The use of this archaic network is both smart and efficient.

Basics:

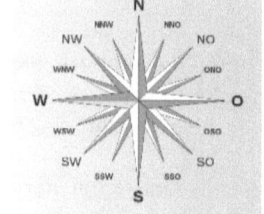 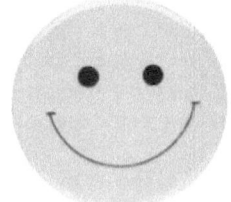

➢ **Face west** (this has better results according to tests done by Dr. Eggetsberger)

➢ **Smile**

➢ **Bend your kness** (flexibility)

➢ **Head up, position:**
   ○ **1st:** **Upright** **better**
   ○ **2nd:** **Sitting** **second choice (**if something is hindering the first choice)

➢ **10 inhalations as a start,** you can increase this later

➢ **All exhalations are matched with contraction of the PC muscle**

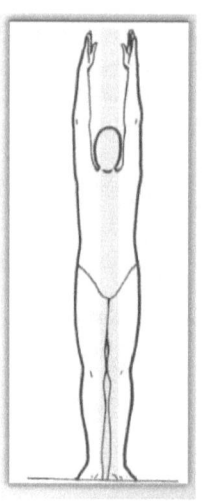

I Rune

The winning pose accelerates a positive mood.
Positive effect on the pituitary, Ajna Chakra (forehead).

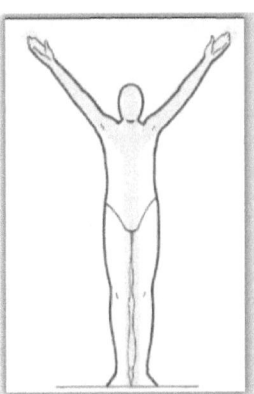

Y Rune

Tension in the upper part of the body => by sheer intuition one is leading to spread and stretch the arms to release tension.

Positive effect on the thyroid, Vishudda Chakra (neck).

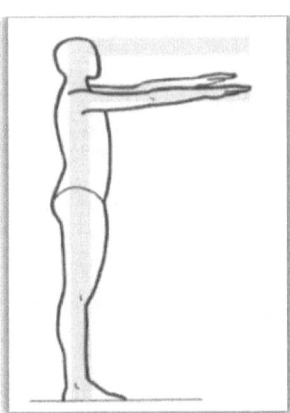

F Rune

Release of tension in the neck and shoulder area.

Positive effect onto the thymus, Anahata Chakra (heart).

Detail: Thumb and mid finger should close the (energy) loop, left arm above right arm!

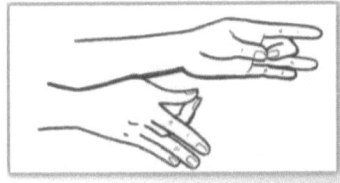

T Rune

Positive effect on the solar plexus, Manipura Chakra (navel).

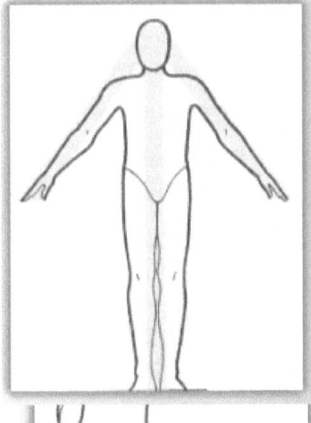

W Rune, dynamic

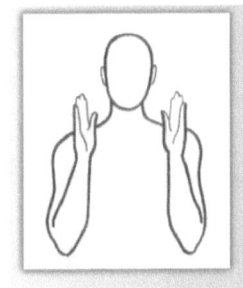

Start by lifting both arms, jerkily throw the left arm to the left. Movement joined with impulsive exhaling.
Repeat with the other arm.

Helps relax the shoulder and neck and releases stress, reduces anxiety and aggression.

= power relax exercise!

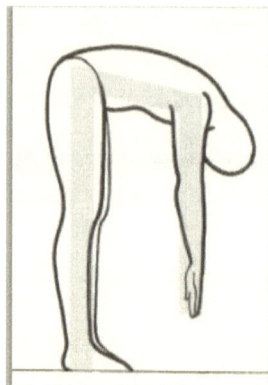

U Rune

Positive effect on the coccyx, Muladhara Chakra.

Opens energy flow from bottom to top. Stretching of the back.

My personal perception:

Input	Output
2 to 3 times per week for 15-20 minutes	Calm mind
	Increased positive attitude
	Flexible spine
	Reduced back Pain
	Stretching of feet
	In the long term, a better body feeling

This is a top leverage exercise. When combined with PC muscle contraction, it's a bit more challenging, and the brain is charged with fresh energy. Whoosh!

If combining both exercises – yoga and PC muscle contraction – your coordination is challenged in a deeper way. This helps in keeping your brain young!

ENERGY FLOW

PHYSIO (Marianne Eder)

Which physiotherapy is right for me?

Marianne Eder

A situation from my practice: A patient visits me for therapy with a package of findings and sinks into the armchair while groaning. My question, "What can I do for you?" is increasingly often answered with an "After the general practitioner, the neurologist and the orthopedic surgeon could no longer help me, it was suggested I try a physiotherapist, a holistic view."

But what is the right therapy, and what is a holistic view?

Our medicine has made fantastic progress. We know more than ever about the body. We can scan and sound it, we can have it depicted from the outside and inside and see all forms that seem to deviate from the norm. But there is also a large field of medicine that functions through experience and emotions, methods that are mostly rationally undetectable, a great field of complementary and alternative medicine - holistic physiotherapy.

Is there a RIGHT method?
When recalling my apprenticeship years as a physiotherapist, many different methods crossed my path. It's important for me to bundle both a variety of therapies together with lot of theory to find the best healing method. The good news is that proven methods to heal do exist.

Evidence-based therapy
For example, if you look at the very common issue of back pain, there is a method here that has been shown to lead to improvement.

1. Coaching
The therapist guides the patient to the appropriate "do-it-yourself technique" to achieve improvement. In the case of back pain, for example, the patient learns to change their posture in as user-friendly a way as possible when standing, sitting and lying down.

Explain Pain Supercharged, David Butler and Lorimer Moseley

Exercise is a master key to your body's medicine cabinet
Exercise is one of the best ways to open the medicine cabinet in your brain. It releases a range of analgesics that are distributed throughout the body. Exercise helps regulate the basic systems that maintain the body's functioning, but which may have become somewhat confused in many persistent pain states. Exercise even promotes the production of anti-inflammatory molecules that calm sensitized hazard sensors and the nerves that relay those hazard signals. But that's not all! Exercise allows you to take on more social activities. It triggers the growth of new brain cells, makes you think better, improves your memory and reaction time, helps you work better and ultimately play better. The point is:

Exercise and training are the best we can do for all our body systems – our cardiovascular system, respiratory system, nerve, hormone and immune systems.
Or the other way around: "Rest = Rust"

2. Proper training

There are a variety of approaches to proper training. Sports scientists around the world fill heavy books in search of optimal training techniques and offer a great spread of ideas. There is no generally accepted valid and correct method.

As a therapist, I pay attention to living conditions, to other basic conditions and to the level of training. **A call for action without overwhelming** the patient is fundamental. Nothing is more frustrating than being overwhelmed, and therapy under strain brings no progress and thus increases frustration.

As a patient, you should do **mild training and sport and increase stepwise**.

If the patient needs more stability due to his clinical picture, stabilizing exercises are the most important. For a lack of mobility, exercises are developed that focus on promoting mobility and stretching. This can, of course, also mean relinquishing certain movements that relieve and heal structures that are injured or inflamed.

For a hobby marathon runner who ambitiously pursues his goal of running for a certain number of hours in half a year, banning running training would require much persuasion and a very good argument.
Pain arises here through a variety of mechanisms:

1. Structures send warning signals (ligaments, muscles, joints, nerves, intervertebral discs, but also intestines, bladder and other organs)
2. Pain sensitivity increases due to psychological mechanisms, e.g. stress, which increase the sensitivity to pain and tension in the muscles
3. Direct or indirect connections of organs and the musculoskeletal system that have a reciprocal influence

Pain? When did it **start, when was it intensified and what was the "quality" of the pain?** Pain can begin quite typically after physical overwork, after a trauma or a fall, in chronic tension, originating from chronic pain-sensitive structures due to inflammation, but also after a long blockage of the intestine and in cases of permanent stress. Very often, intervertebral discs, joints and the muscles in this area hurt, but the intestines or organs can also set the pain spiral in motion.
I also find the connections between the intestine and the musculoskeletal system very exciting. These connections have only recently become more of a focus.

The **intestines and organs have fascial compounds** with the musculoskeletal system, but even through proximity and the same supply through nerves, back pain can arise which can cause a pronounced blockage of the intestine, perhaps through malnutrition. Also, permanent stress increases the tone in the smooth muscles of the intestine, which then causes tension pain and negatively affects the peristalsis (movement) of the intestine. This, in turn, leads to constipation ... the pain spiral is starting to turn!

Therefore, the medical history of the patient should also include questions about nutrition and stool behavior because this also affects the development of pain.

Thus, in addition to **movement behavior and posture**, both the diet and **mental health and stress** have an impact on overcoming the pain.

Healing takes time! Healing resurrects the body

Franz: How did Marianne treat my injuries? She dealt with my problems with a great amount of skill:

1. A twice-broken left arm resulting from my clumsy driving of a motocross bike in a training course. The short-term idea was learning to drive. The long-term vision behind the scene was a solid mid-life crisis pulling me into perilous waters. I blame myself.

2. Neck tension due to high stress in my job. Once again, I blame myself – I could have learnt to deal with the stress better, for example by breathing away the tension and the stress.

3. Problems with my shoulders. In fact, it was supraspinatus tendinitis. The big tendon joining the upper arm muscle with my shoulder was abraded and the bone structure showed signs of abrasion. A small cyst increased the pain and reduced leverage.
I detected this when doing my Sunday morning exercises for spinal training. "Oh, the right shoulder sucks!" An orthopedic doctor said it was "like a frayed thong."

Healing needs time and I had to suffer again for the greater good of regaining agility!

1.) A special bandage fixed my left arm to my body for about six weeks. This helped the broken bones to reconnect with the price being reduced agility (by more than 90%) in the shoulder. Although incredible to believe, the shoulder was practically stiff!
In short, oscillation of the left arm upwards and sideward increased slowly by moving the joint under strict supervision.

2.) The neck and shoulder were stiff and far too tense. Sound familiar in this high-stress world?
   ⇨ **Head up** was the first advice from Marianne. Somehow, I had incorporated the smartphone looking-downwards behavior.
   ⇨ Put a towel around your neck and **bend your head back.** This is not a very sophisticated technique, but for this reason it easy to remember and to include in your daily routine.
   ⇨ **Raise your shoulders as high as possible and let them fall with gravity.**

You can follow the rest of the exercises for the neck and the shoulders in my download section.

STRESS
(Markus Eggetsberger)

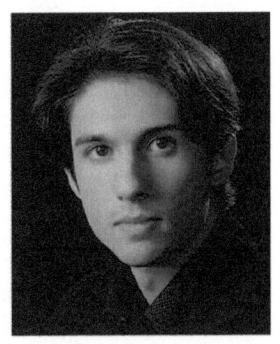

Our body is regulated by two nervous systems: the sympathetic and parasympathetic nervous systems. At rest, both are in balance. As soon as they become imbalanced – as stress arises – they try to rebalance themselves. Classical stress reactions are attributed to the two nervous systems. The sympathetic nervous system is the arousing nervous system. Sympathetic responses usually correspond to "classic stress responses." These include nervousness, anger, escape reactions or blushing. In contrast, the stress responses of the parasympathetic nervous system are often overlooked. These include subtler reactions such as nausea, solidification or even circulatory problems.

By nature, every person prefers to respond to stress with one of these two "stress systems." This is innate, and each predisposition offers its own pros and cons.

From the outside world, parasympathetic often seem very calm and controlled. However, their stress symptoms are often delayed and invisible to many observers. Basically, it is important to understand that for each of the two reactions, the opposite represents the regulatory counterpoint. This means that after every tantrum (the sympathetic nervous system) there must always be a dampening (the parasympathetic nervous system). With particularly strong reactions – a strong tantrum – equally strong regulatory backlashes will result. The strong cushioning of the parasympathetic nervous system can thus be perceived by sufferers as "exhaustion" after the tantrum. If one continues to follow the course of such a reaction, the sympathetic would now (more gently) counteract. This happens repeatedly until a relatively balanced state arises. The balancing of the sympathetic nervous system and parasympathetic nervous system therefore represents our actual state of relaxation.

This can be illustrated simply in the example of our breathing. Every inhalation is a sympathetic reaction (arousal) and every exhalation is a reaction of the parasympathetic nervous system (cushioning). Thus, calm breathing could have a breathing ratio of 1:1. Keeping our nervous system in mind, this means that equal parts are aroused as well as dampened. This creates a natural and healthy balance between the two nervous systems.

In this balanced and stress-free state, our brain, especially the consciously thinking and crucial areas of the frontal lobe, have the best preconditions for best performance. A modern relaxation concept should therefore not contain general relaxation exercises for "every human being," as such a thing can only work to a limited extent. You should recognize your own reactions and learn which type of nervous system you correspond with and thus orient your life accordingly.

If I am a nervous and **choleric sympathetic**, it is advantageous for me to learn to dampen myself (parasympathetic nervous system) to avoid overreactions and reduced performance. An example of such a measure could be the "**1:4 breathing**." The 1:4 stands for the respiratory ratio. From the statement above, we know that compensation could be found at approximately 1:1. In a ratio of 1:4, the parasympathetic nervous system, which is the cushioning, is stimulated four times as much as the sympathetic nervous system that produces the arousal. So, it's easy to understand that by repeatedly performing this 1:4 breathing, the nervous system can move from an increased sympathetic reaction back to a more equal state.

What applies to the sympathetic is, of course, also a reality for a **parasympathetic** nervous system person. However, this is prone to over-absorption and should always ensure a **good basic activity**! A tailor-made relaxation training that respects the prevailing types of nerves is a very good investment in one's health and performance. It is also important to note that if stress is ignored for too long and, above all, if a permanent stress state is reached, the result will be increased anxiety. The limbic system and the amygdalae (fear center) within it always recognize long-term and permanent stress as a cause for anxiety.

Franz: I found through Dr Eggetsberger research, with lots of cables on my head, that I'm the parasympathetic type who should preferably do basic activities to accelerate.

Learn something about the Eggetsberger work and tremendous experience:

https://www.biovitshop.com/

https://www.facebook.com/EggetsbergerNET-233950591657/

RELAX

Mankind has landed on the moon, fired missiles into deep space to explore the interstellar room, built quantum-based computers and is increasing the lifespan of mankind to overcome decay and death. AI and robots are on the brink of helping (and replacing?) mankind.

Brave new world, or still captive in the Stone Age, eye to eye with the dangerous sabre-toothed tiger?

What is the sabre-toothed Tiger these days?

- Losing a job, a partner, your health or being unproductive in this oh-so productive world.
- Loss of life savings resulting from a world crisis – remember the crash of Lehman Brothers!
- Or simply getting older (and not being stuffed with the right funds).
- Cyber security flows away because imposters break into data storage which results in no privacy and blackmailing as the likely outcomes.
- Losing connection with our "friends" in this superficial world of social networks.
- Disastrous climate conditions.
- Gladiatorial activities between the great players in the world.
- Or simply all the bad news on TV and social media intruding into our lives, producing fear in everybody and making it easier for us to be manipulated.

Distraction:
The daily consumption of huge amounts of new information (mostly bad) intrudes in our lives and is increasingly bad for our calmness. We are always on alert via e-mail. Mobile phones have merged with arms and ears – observe this addictive behaviour on public transport or in a restaurant. Are we web-addicts?

I visited the island Stromboli some 10 years ago and again last year. On the first visit it was easy to connect with people and it was not so crowded. On my last visit there were more people and they were "merged" with their smart phones leaving little room for encounters – a loss of communication.

What are the possible reactions when a person is in great danger (attack of the sabre-toothed tiger!):

- Flee   =   (shit and) run
- Play dead   =   shock, no movement, brain is a flat liner
- Fight

These patterns are etched deeply into our limbic systems, the domicile of a very old part of our brain. The problem is not a once-off avoidance of danger but a chronicled stress situation – again and again and again. This changes a lot in our body, just like a bad influence in our digestive system (constipation or diarrhea) which itself disempowers the immune system, blocks the blood vessels, disturbs sleep and increases the risk of diabetes and fat storage (the deposit for bad times).

Tension in the muscles which are a shell to protect us against the bad things around us, steals our energy which cannot flow steadily and easily but is blocked. There is too much energy somewhere in the body and somewhere else there is too little energy. This means an imbalanced body and, as a result, an imbalanced mind.

Conclusion – stress is THE enemy!

My problems are constipation and a stiff neck!

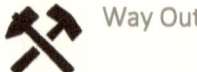 Way Out

⇨ **Reduce telephone use (**especially in the evening, because sleep will improve)
⇨ **Reduce e-mail use**
⇨ **Perfection isn't a must**
⇨ **Go out into nature, take a walk**
⇨ **Express your feelings**
⇨ **Soft thyroid massage, especially as you get older**

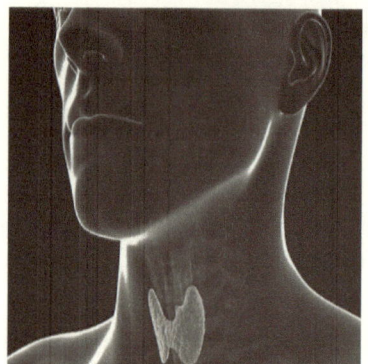

Positive effects of a soft thyroid massage are:

- Increased willpower, better mood
- Higher basal metabolic rate (fat burner)
- Also: it's getting warmer!
- Higher resilience against stress
- Anti-inflammatory effect
- Strengthens bones
- Lowers blood fat

All in all – more power

With the index finger and thumb, softly massage the thyroid 50-100x, change the massaging hands. Paradoxically, this works even before sleep.

⇨ **1:4 breathing exercise**; this means 1 unit inhalation and 4 units exhalation. The theory: 1 unit sympathetic and 4 units parasympathetic. The latter provides relaxation. As your skill improves, increase this stepwise to 1:11. Breathing is for free, use it!

Breath all tension in the body away with gentle moaning. I do this when my back pain is tough, or my neck is too hard. With every breath, I focus on these parts and softly sigh the pain away. The sound is an "om" or a deep "ah," which better connects you to the universe and eases the pain in the body. "Ah" is often automatically produced if you have pain. The pain is reduced by the body emitting interleukin-2, which is like aspirin. Thus, om or ah
⇨ creates vibrations in the whole body. This is good for improved energy flow, especially in the spinal cord.

If your breath is steady and slow (6 cycles per minute), the brain only requires a very low energy input, which is an optimum situation. This technique has been practiced over millennia in yoga and meditation. Maybe this effect was discovered through exercise – without using any measuring instruments. It is like going back some 10,000 years or more in the development of the human brain.

Slow breathing can reduce anxiety, stress and pain!

I once told my mother that mankind was still living in the Stone Age or somewhere else far behind our modern time schedule. Civilization is just a modern suit and a small tremor could shake it all apart! She didn't believe this, but it was obvious to me. I insist on the fact that modern mankind is still captivated in ancient times.

This means:
Accepting this ancient track record – our development from former times is worth considering. I feel quite comfortable in looking into the open fire in the evening when the firewood is burning in the oven or sitting around the fireplace and discussing the events of the day or the plans for tomorrow with the group of people I love to be with. Feeling at home, finding some sort of a root in life that often tends to be without roots and steady anchors!

Why not include ancient wisdom in our daily life?

⇨ **Feel the pulsation in your fingertips – or pray.**

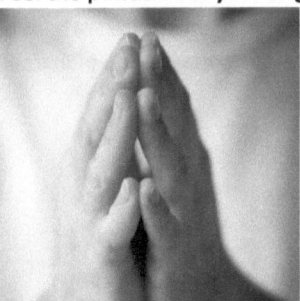

The positive effects are:
- Tension decreases
- Blood vessels extend themselves
- Hands become warmer, and pulse rate is lowered
- Headaches or even light migraines can disappear
- Greater calmness
- Consciousness for the body grows

The theory behind this is that the **mind can focus on one issue only**: either it focuses on its sorrows or it **feels the pulsation** ☺
Choose wisely.

⇨ **PCE muscle training to increase brain activity.**

⇨ **Jacobsen's muscle relaxation training, to decrease basic tension in your muscles.**

⇨ **Meditation:** If you aren't skilled in meditation techniques – no problem.
Just sit still and straight for some minutes and think of NOTHING!
Extend this time to 5 or 10 minutes a day.
If thoughts come, let them pass.
Concentrate on your slow, gentle breath and focus on your fontanel.

Move down the spine from one cycle of inhalation to the next cycle of inhalation to the bottom of the spine, then move up again to the fontanel.

A wise man once said the following about the duration:
On normal Days: 20 min.
On stressful days where time is short: 60 min.

Meditation is the only exercise you can never ever do too much of!

"Because I've heard it's good for the health, I've decided to be happy" Paul Watzlawick.

Sogyal Rinpoche states in his book:
The Tibetan Book of Living and Dying.

"To learn meditation correctly is the greatest gift you can give yourself. By meditation you can find the true Nature of yourself. Only within Meditation you can find Stability and Trust you need to live and die in a good way. Meditation is the way to enlightenment."

He also says that there should be great trust between master and disciple. From this, exercises will be understood in good time and will not be unnecessarily delayed. He also gives a very important piece of basic advice: look for the LINE of your master. This means that if you know who the predecessor of your master was and who passed this honor on to your master, you can your trust that the wisdom and knowledge was learned and passed to the next generation for the greater good.

If someone stands alone with his honor, he has most likely inaugurated himself – pope and imperator in one person. This is most likely a charlatan and not a good guru or friend, and there are a lot of them crowding our soil. Their benefit is your money flowing into their pockets instead of increasing your spiritual development.

Take care and choose wisely. **Lookout for the line!**

I feel very fortunate in finding this source of wisdom described very practically by Sogyal Rinpoche. Take your time studying his book, you'll not regret it!

Considering death as real will make life more real. And then life will be used in a better way.

"*The word yoga is derived from the Sanskrit root yuj, which means to join. The science of Kriya yoga teaches the method of merging the individual will with the cosmic will by controlling the mind and its modifications, thereby attaining liberation. On the physical plane, yoga bestows good health and physical efficiency; on the mental plane concentration, balance of mind and peace. On the spiritual plane, it guarantees liberation from the chain of birth and death and offers eternal bliss, immortality, perfection and everlasting peace. The ultimate objective of yoga is not only individual liberation but the transformation of the entire human race. It aims to instill a divine nature and life into the physical, mental and spiritual life of humanity. Yoga has several branches, but Kriya Yoga is the essence of all yoga's.*"

- - - *Paramahamsa Hariharananda Maharaj* - - -

Frequencies out of the Eggetsberger Box.

These frequencies aren't about the movie. No, these are little helpers from the Bio-Vit Shop to increase brain activity and decrease anxiety. They are stepwise development tools.

Neurostick, 27 Frequencies   It starts with Alpha giving peace, further increasing tact, opening your mind, increasing energy levels and comes to om which, for unknown reasons, synchronizes the left and right brain hemispheres to arrive at a relaxed coolness which both relaxes and strengthens the brain. **With OM I can even do difficult Sodukos** – mysterious, but the effect is clear.

When you delve into these frequencies you'll have to ask Dr Google for help because all the descriptions are in German. The actual frequencies are international – no specific language ☺ Just frequencies.

Better self-awareness With this, you can increase love, find and explore potential talents and stimulate intelligence.

I found lot of other helpful tools developed by Dr Eggetsberger and his family. It is important for him that his trainees understand the concept and the theory behind his inventions. Together with this knowledge, one can practice alone. Look here for more inspiration: *Dr Gerhard Eggetsberger* (translator recommended).
I also use some additional gadgets, but these are connected to relevant training courses, so you won't get them just by clicking through the web shop without attending the training course.

My girlfriend sometimes chuckles about my mild addiction to these gadgets, but I believe that in the long run they are helpful in strengthening the mind and soul.

Power injector for cellular energy This tool increases the power level within the cells.

Toolbox Against Stress and Bad Moods and When I'm Angry
⇨ 1:4 breathing; extend to 1:11 and switch slowly to the energy centers
⇨ Feel your pulse; I also do this in business meetings (under the table in order not to arouse suspicion ☺)
⇨ PCE muscle training
⇨ Listen to frequencies
⇨ Soft thyroid massage in the car

Toolbox Against Worrying Thoughts:
⇨ Stop breathing for a moment
⇨ Ask yourself: Who am I?
⇨ Ask yourself: What is my next thought?

Toolbox for Positive Emotions:
⇨ Stare into space   =   stop thinking
⇨ Smile, especially on the left side   =   happy
⇨ Toes up like a baby   =   happy
⇨ Concentrate on the solar plexus   =   now

⇨ Each time you drink a glass of water think: **"The world is in peace, and I am too."** According to quantum physics, these thoughts produce high-frequency vibrations towards peace. Repeat and repeat and share the thinking and it will grow.

Negative or positive stress (one coin, two sides)

Life without sense	Life with sense
No direction, no goal	Difficulty is easier to bear
No schedule	Increased responsibility

| Loss of sense | Better relaxation |
| Burnout is near | Better health |

I found that setting clear goals gave my life direction. The little and many gadgets I have tried and still try are, to some extent, simple play tools for a grown-up boy – they shouldn't be taken too seriously.

NATURE
(Sibylle Steidl)

Nature-assisted therapy – a simple forest walk is good medicine

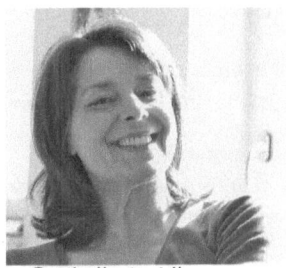

© Sibylle Steidl

Anyone who likes to walk in the forest knows that the grey life flies away when hiking in the woods. It just feels good to wander beneath the canopy of leaves, breathing in the spicy air and weighing in with the rhythm of your steps.

This truism is scientifically backed up with facts: **The forest keeps us healthy, it animates us and is healing!** In a recent study, the American scientist, Mary Carol R. Hunter of the University of Michigan and her team, found that after a forest walk lasting just 20 minutes, the body's stress hormone cortisol is significantly lowered. *Link to the study*

In plain language, this means that those who regularly walk in the forest remain calm and balanced, even in difficult life situations. This, in turn, has an extremely beneficial effect on blood pressure, the heart, circulation, digestion, sleep quality, concentration and personal mood.

Cortisol, together with other stress hormones such as adrenaline and norepinephrine, causes the body to rise to peak performance under stress in the short term. In terms of evolution, stress is a reaction to – often supposed – danger. To escape this, our brains switch to "flight" or "fight." These are basic routines working in the reptile part of the brain – an unconscious reaction in the blink of an eye. The body's own drug cocktail, consisting of cortisol and other stress hormones, also ensures that we can react and run faster, feel strong and feel neither pain nor hunger.

However, the pendulum can turn the other way if you are exposed to this hormonal blast in the long term. It starts with sleep problems, which in turn increase stress hormones, resulting in the beginning of a devil's cycle. The consequences can hurt both body and soul. This includes cardiovascular problems, high blood pressure, tension, musculoskeletal damage, digestive difficulties and pain. Mental impairments include difficulty concentrating, memory, anxiety, depression and burnout.

To escape this downward spiral, a **simple daily walk in the forest helps**. In Japan, for this reason, the concept of "forest bathing" for stricken Japanese city-dwellers was launched. In five forest communication centers, the Japanese learn to practice idleness between the trees, to consciously breathe, to rest and to discover slowness. Under the leadership of the Japanese researcher, university professor and deputy director of the Center for Environment, Health and Field Research at the University of Chiba, Yoshifumi Miyazaki, this medically tested forest lingering is used as a medically prescribed therapy. Meanwhile, more than five million Japanese enjoy the refreshing air under the canopy of leaves.

The healing and regenerating effect of nature in general and specifically that of trees is nothing new. Even our ancestors knew about the power of the trees. A village had its **village tree** around which meetings and gatherings took place, and the myths and fairy tales of the forest often played an important role. In the 1970s, the evolutionary biologist, Edward O. Wilson, explored the healing interaction between humans and nature in his work *Biophilia*. He was convinced that nature is the essence of life and therefore also that humans have an inherent "love for all living things."

Quod erat demonstrandum!

Four simple exercises that help you rest in the forest, sharpen your senses, allow freshness to flow into your thinking and improve calmness.

1.   **Spontaneously find a tree.**
        Stand at ten meters and consciously perceive its shape. Has it just grown or is it curved? Where does it grow? In which direction does it point? Is it very branched or more linear? Can you smell the resins, hear the leaves rustling, see what the light looks like through the green thicket ...?

        Let the tree work on you by spreading your arms and welcoming it.

        Now look for a place under the tree. Stare vacantly up into the crown, free of any intention. Concentrate on your breath. Watch your breath and let the energy of the tree affect you. Spend about 15 minutes doing this.

2.   **Stand up and lean on the tree with your back**.
        Continue to breath consciously.

        Feel the inside of your body. Where are the blockages, tension or pain? Pass them over to the tree. In the process, imagine how the tree absorbs all its fears, stress and tension and transforms all of this to release fresh, pure oxygen.
        Breathe consciously.

3.   **Walk ahead and slow your pace**.
        Slow it again. And again. Now, at every step, perceive the soil under your feet.
        Is it hard or soft? Do you feel the roots, stones or leaves?

        Feel the shift in body weight with every step you take. From the right hip to the left and vice versa. Do this for about ten minutes.

4.   **Slow your pace again.**
        Consciously perceive your surroundings. Smell the scent of the forest, feel a branch lying on the ground, hear the singing of the birds, perceive the different shades of green in the forest. Walk ahead and focus entirely on your perception.
        You and the forest are one.

Sibylle Steidl

Psychotherapist, hiking guide, environmental activist and artist

© Copyright 2019, Sibylle Steidl, Gars am Kamp, Austria

REPOSITORY

Hiking

Put both feet on the ground:

- **Parallel** – your knees will thank you very much when you grow old.
- **Have full contact with the ground** and don't dance around like a ballerina on only your toes. <u>Toes only means less stability.</u>

Always take, as a minimum, light **gloves and a cap** with you. You'll be happy to have this protection for your hands in rocky areas and for your head from the sun.

- GoPro with arm mount and voice control – both arms are free
- Adjustable walking sticks as a "4X4" for both directions.
    - Up: more power
    - Down: protection of knees and joints
- If you have glasses, use contact lenses (day lenses can be used for up to two days).
- Small power-bank to increase the range of your mobile phone.
- Functional sportswear to increase your time range without needing to carry too many additional clothes for a few days. Two to three days' worth is enough and has the advantage of a lighter load!
- Toothbrush for the night(s).
- Headlight. Provided you Mobile has enough energy this could be skipped.

Travelling

Reduce your luggage to a minimum:

- Boarding case or backpack with 8 kg as the goal.
- Bike backpack as handbag.
- Empty liquid bottle to refill with water after check in.
- Compression socks, if needed, for longer flights to avoid thrombosis.
  Always drink a lot of water on the plane.
- Small headphones.
- Scarf as a mini pillow.
- Mini toilette package: one razor blade, aftershave in reduced travel size, laundry detergent (or use the laundry service in the hotel).
- Bay slippers for the room and the bay.
- Take and leave old worn out clothes and replace with new items as a type of souvenir. I've a Cinque Terre shirt at home which reminds me of a lovely time there.
- Functional clothes could be worn in two sizes (long or short).
- Gifts to be sent home by post or courier.

NEW

Don't be too critical of yourself, learn new things and explore new paths like a child learning the very basics. Improvement and extension of wisdom will follow naturally.

As a kid you learnt slowly and made some mistakes. These didn't bother you then. Every time you failed at the first step, you got up again. So, stand up young kid ☺ It's never too late. Life is a BIG learning session.

I'll never forget the first horseshoe I made at my friend's blacksmith. A retired blacksmith saw my poor attempt, more like an alien shoe than a horseshoe, took it by forceps, held it up to the bright light and asked me: "Have you ever seen such a horse?" Great laughter!

And I wanted to crawl into the ground :-(

This experienced blacksmith skillfully struck the shoe a few times and the alien shoe miraculously turned into a beautiful horseshoe. Lesson learned: Don't give in so easily when doing new things. They are new for everyone. Be patient with the "kid" inside yourself. I gained experience with many years of practice and my works are now good for me personally or are fine gifts, bringing joy to me and my friends: horseshoes, a violin clef, an om sign, a candleholder, Saint Francis within the birds sermon, a hook to attach big flower pots, handrails, a drinking trough for birds, etc. If my vision didn't prevail, all these awesome things wouldn't have been born. I was even once asked if I was a smith doing art – wow, that rocked!

"A small spark could lead to a big fire" and "Man forges his own destiny."

Formula 1 world champion Niki Lauda said simply when encouraging people to try new ways:
"DO IT!"

Matts Mullenweg Opens His Bag
This constantly travelling man shows us a lot on how to be efficient when travelling.

My Movie List

Title	Year	Director	Type	Intro
Master and Commander	2003	Peter Weir	Action, Adventure, Drama	Russel Crowe showed signs of mastery as an actor. A strong leader overcoming a weakness in gear in a fight with a far better enemy.
Arn, the Knight Templar	2010	Peter Flinth	Action, Adventure, Drama	Arn must endure so much before he can get the love of his life, Cecilie, who has been put away in a monastery. Take your time for this 4-hour marathon.
King Artur	2004	Antoine Fuqua	Action, Adventure, Drama	A strong movie of King Arthur and the Knights of the Round Table, thanks to an excellent cast: Keira Knightley, Clive Owen, Ioan Gruffudd, Mads Mikkelsen, Stellan Skarsgard, Til Schweiger, etc.
Doctor Strange	2016	Scott Derrickson	Action, Adventure, Fantasy	A brilliant and arrogant neurosurgeon faces helplessness. By stepping into the world of the mystic arts somewhere in Nepal he discovers great and, thus far, hidden skills within himself. Great Benedict Cumberbatch, who started in theatre before he changed to movies.
A Knight's Tale	2001	Brian Helgeland	Action, Adventure, Romance	William Thatcher (Heath Ledger) is rearranging his stars following his father's advice. Count Adhemar (Rufus Sewell) is a good counterpart to Thatcher.

TRON	1982	Steven Linsberger	Action, Adventure, Sci-Fi	A computer hacker is sucked into a digital world facing a hostile new world. Due to changes in our world from analog to digital this story is a detailed prediction of what is to come. Jeff Bridges is as good as ever.
Point Break	1991	Katheryn Bigelow	Action, Crime, Thriller	In my eyes, Patrick Swayze's best performance ever. Keanu Reeves was always behind and was somehow addicted to Bodhi. The spell was broken by love!
Vantage Point	2008	Pete Travis	Action, Crime, Drama	The attempted assassination of the American president is told from eight different perspectives. Changing perspective helps change the point of view: The world is not only black and white, it is sometimes grey and sometimes correct is incorrect from another's viewpoint.
The Matrix	1999	Lana and Lilly Wachovsky	Action, Sci-Fi	What would you think if your whole life was just a lie? Would you take the red (awakening life with its many troubles and possibilities) or the blue (continuation) pill?
The Gold Rush	1925	Charlie Chaplin (also stars)	Adventure, Comedy, Drama	A gold prospector goes to the Klondike in search of gold and finds it … and much more.
Seven Samurai	1954	Akiro Kurosawa	Adventure, Drama	A poor village under attack by bandits recruits seven unemployed samurai to help them defend themselves. Toshiro Mifune was the teacher in martial arts and the strategist against the treacherous thieves.
White Squall	1996	Ridley Scott	Adventure, Drama	Teenage boys discover discipline and camaraderie on an ill-fated sailing voyage. Jeff Bridges is a strong captain forming young men.
Artificial Intelligence: AI	2001	Steven Spielberg	Adventure, Drama, Sci-Fi	A highly advanced robotic boy longs to become "real" so that he can regain the love of his human mother. A precise forecast of what is going on right now. Osment played the character seeking a mother's love very convincingly.
Turning Tide	2013	Christophe Offenstein	Adventure, Drama, Sport	Yann Kermadec started a round-the-world non-stop single-handed yacht race. After several days of racing, in the lead, Yann must stop to repair a damaged rudder. This will disrupt his round-the-world journey … A very tough Francois Cluzet facing the elements.

Title	Year	Director	Type	Intro
Rush	2013	Ron Howard	Action. Biography, Drama	The Austrian legend Niki Lauda's rivalry against his big Formula 1 rival James Hunt (GB). Finally, the emotions switched. Energy, love, tragedy and comradeship. Both actors good or even outstanding.
The Intouchables	2011	Olivier Nakache, Éric Toledano	Biography, Comedy, Drama	After he becomes a quadriplegic in a paragliding accident, an aristocrat hires a young man from the projects to be his caregiver. Omar Sy and Francois Cluzet are outstanding. Friends in real life.
Green Book	2018	Peter Farrelly	Biography, Drama	Theoretical intellect (an African American pianist) meets practical intellect (an Italian American bouncer) on a journey through racism in the 1960s, when hate was everywhere. Finally, both antagonists became lifelong friends.
First Man	2018	Damien Chazelle	Biography, Drama, History	A look at the life of the astronaut, Neil Armstrong, and the legendary space mission that led him to become the first man to walk on the moon on July 20, 1969. At the age of eight, I followed every step of this great adventure that entered a new world – the moon. Neil Armstrong was a real warhorse, keeping cool when fire was all around him.
The King's Speech	2010	Tom Hooper	Biography, Drama, History	Colin Firth (King George VI) trained by Geoffrey Rush (a speech therapist) in overcoming his speech disability. Very unusual training methods, but effective in overcoming the stammer. The crowd finally respected their new King
Chasing Mavericks	2012	Michael Apted, Curtis Hanson	Biography, Drama, Sport	When young Jay Moriarty discovers that the mythic Mavericks surf break, one of the biggest waves on earth, exists just miles from his Santa Cruz home, he enlists the help of local legend Frosty Hesson to train him to survive it. Gerald Butler nearly died on the set (in a big wave).

Title	Year	Director	Type	Intro
The Great Race	1965	Blake Edwards	Comedy	In the early 20th century, two rivals, the heroic Leslie and the despicable Professor Fate, engage in an epic automobile race from New York to Paris. Great performance by Jack Lemmon
Bonnie Scotland	2035	James W. Horne	Comedy	Stan Laurel and Oliver Hardy join the army and find themselves posted to the North-West Frontier in India on a dangerous mission. The plan was to get a free new suit.
The Party	1968	Blake Edwards	Comedy	Peter Sellers causing chaos at an exclusive Hollywood party is historic and fun from the very first moment.
Planes, Trains and Automobiles	1987	John Hughes	Comedy	A man must struggle to travel home for Thanksgiving with a shower curtain ring salesman as his only companion. John Candy and Steve Martin on probably their funniest winter journey back home.
Welcome to the Sticks	2008	Jan Seemann	Comedy	A post office director was punished and sent to the "freezing" cold north of France. His first trip by car was stunningly funny: police suggested he step on the accelerator. Seems like he didn't want to go up north. But things changed ….
The Naked Gun	1988	David Zucker	Comedy, Crime	The ever great Leslie Nielsen performing superbly in comedy. Stumbling from one error to the next and finally doing something good.
Dr. Strangelove or: How I Learned to Stop Worrying and Love the Bomb	1964	Stanley Kubrick	Comedy, Drama	An insane general trigger a path to nuclear holocaust that a war room full of politicians and generals frantically try to stop. Peter Sellers shows his great acting skills outside of comedy with Stanley Kubrick revealing his genius!
The Concert	2009	Radu Mihaileanu	Comedy, Drama, Music	Music is the basic transporter for passion, love and … old secrets. Tears of pain and joy exchange places within short course. Creativity and a long-buried dream were helped to fly up into the sky. Project business at its best.
As it is in Heaven	2004	Kay Pollak	Comedy, Drama, Music	A successful international conductor had a burnout and had to recover in a quiet place – his childhood village in the very north of Sweden. He soon started as the master of the church choir, unleashing energy in the members that they had never before experienced. But every action has a reaction, and problems arose. Music is again the transporter of passion and love. Michael Nyquist as actor finds his Swedish roots.

Grumpy Old Men	1993	Donald Petrie	Comedy, Drama, Romance	Two elderly neighbors became even more unfriendly towards each other when trying to win a woman, but finally conceded in friendship. Burgess Meredith's comments on the time for sex between a man and woman were very funny! In real life, Walter Matthau and Jack Lemmon used to be best friends!
A Good Year	2006	Ridley Scott	Comedy, Drama, Romance	A British investment broker inherits his uncle's chateau and vineyard in Provence, where he spent much of his childhood. He discovers a new laid-back lifestyle as he tries to renovate the estate for sale. A romantic work of art from Ridley Scott who owns a house in Provence in real life. Russel Crowe in a non-martial arts movie – rare!
Life is Beautiful	1997	Roberto Benigni (also stars)	Comedy, Drama, Romance	When an open-minded Jewish librarian and his son become victims of the Holocaust, he uses a perfect mixture of will, humor and imagination to protect his son from the dangers around their camp.
Sweet Home Alabama	2002	Andy Tennant	Comedy, Romance	Reese Witherspoon had to resolve old problems at home in Alabama. She learned her lesson: Don't forget Mama and Papa when a career call! Lynard Skynyrd produced the soundtrack.
A Clockwork Orange	1971	Stanley Kubrick	Crime, Drama, Sci-Fi	In the future, a sadistic gang leader is imprisoned and must undergo a counter action experiment. But it doesn't go as planned.
Planet Earth II	2016	David Attenborough	Documentary	David Attenborough returns in this breathtaking documentary showcasing life on Planet Earth.

Title	Year	Director	Type	Intro
Gran Torino	2008	Clint Eastwood	Drama	A Korean War veteran, Walt Kowalski, sets out to reform his neighbor, a teenager who tried to steal Kowalski's prized possession – a 1972 Gran Torino. The elderly Clint Eastwood is amazingly outstanding. An ideal image of how one (me?) should perform in old age. Look out for "The Mule."
K-19	2002	Kathryn Bigelow	Drama, History, Thriller	The disaster – Russia's first nuclear submarine malfunctions – happened in 1961, my year of birth. The world was on the brink of a war – and I was happy in my cradle, unconscious of the things around me. The very first captain's test of his ship and crew to its limits was fierce. Slowly the whole crew understood why – knowing the borders.
Enemy at the Gates	2001	Jean-Jacques Annaud	Drama, History, War	A Russian and a German sniper play a game of cat-and-mouse during the Battle of Stalingrad. Top performance by Jude Law (the Russian sniper) and Ed Harris (the German sniper)
The English Patient	1996	Anthony Minghella	Drama, Romance	At the end of WWII, a young nurse tends to a badly burned plane crash victim. His past is shown in flashbacks, revealing an involvement in a fateful love affair. Combining the lovely countryside of Italy with the endless horizons of the Sahara Desert, it is easy to understand the positive image of the movie. This gentle picture came to a sudden halt when a bomb dismantling team carefully tries to disarm a bomb and a tank shakes and rattles the entire soil around the specialists.
Rain Man	1988	Barry Levinson	Drama, Romance	Selfish yuppie Charlie Babbitt's father left a fortune to his savant brother Raymond and a pittance to Charlie; they travel cross-country. My elder brother was savant too, so this is a kind of recall of life. Dustin Hoffman's performance is extraordinary.
My Summer in Provence	2014	Rose Bosch	Drama, Romance	Lea, Adrian and their little brother Theo, born deaf, go on holiday in Provence with their grandfather. They never met because of a family quarrel. Unfortunately, it is not the holiday they dreamed of. In less than 24 hours, there is a clash of generations between the teens and their grandfather. Jean Reno was the grumpy old grandpa only in the beginning …
Gravity	2013	Alfonso Cuaron	Drama, Sci-Fi, Thriller	Two astronauts work together to survive after an accident leaves them stranded in space. Stunning pictures of earth seen from space, debris, fear on the brink of "to be or not to be" and then human creativity solves the puzzle. Sandra Bullock's embryonic position is vivid!
Fearless	1993	Peter Weir	Drama, Thriller	A man starts a new life after surviving an airline crash. Jeff Bridges is brilliant as ever!

The Hurt Locker	2008	Kathryn Bigelow	Drama, Thriller, War	A Sergeant is assigned to an army bomb squad with his squad mates. Tension from the very beginning! Jeremy Renner's lift off as a movie star.
Thin Red Line	1998	Terrence Malick	Drama, War	Adaptation of James Jones' autobiographical 1962 novel focusing on the conflict at Guadalcanal during the Second World War. Pictures of great beauty changed into pictures of destruction. Terence Malick productions are rare and good.

Alone

In modern (western) times people are crowded by people and filled with lots of impressions. This only leaves a small space for quietness. It is as if calmness is to be avoided and crowding is the goal. People who are not connected to their inner self are easier to control and manipulate. Don't expect any help for from the top for calmness within yourself.

Disruption or Helper:

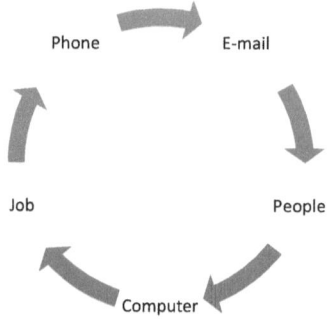

This spinning wheel is turning fast and loud. There is no place for quietness and time for reflection or to listen to the inner voice of what is good or not good for oneself.

To be alone – e.g. on a walk in the forest or on a hiking tour – is important as it provides time to listen to the inner self without any disruptions from the outside. I have figured out that major decisions need space and time to be reflected upon without disturbance.

I do this through:

- Walking or hiking   regularly
- A vacation week alone   once a year
- A retreat in a camp   once a year

Doing this requires some courage to feel at home with yourself alone. If everything causing trouble is systematically removed, only the inner self remains. Then the moment of truth is near – what is within?

These steps require courage because reflection could be with nothing or with something new. It could imply the need for a change of perception, a change of habits. And change requires some effort. Staying in the world of consumption is far easier.

Book List

Some moving books I have already mentioned. The rest is available in German only.

I trust Tim Ferris' book list and would, most humbly, like to refer to the book lists of

Bill Gates or *Richard Branson*.

CASH

I'm not a skilled broker and switch frequently during the day from one value to another. I have a university degree in accounting and have held the position of finance manager for more than 30 years. My behavior is conservative. I'm far too slow for trading. My strengths are as a good analyst and evaluator of opportunities and risks and saving money in the long-term range. I could have been a good sniper! Listening to and reading about experienced persons is a must for me.

Forward-looking is maybe the best description of this strength. I don't have access to deep analysis systems which could figure out good or bad rumors earlier for me than for others. Remember the crash of Lehman Brothers in 2008 was obvious half a month prior to the crash …

Older Patterns from Childhood
1. Bank account, or savings account
2. Saving money in building societies
3. Life insurance
4. Real estate

Everything is combined in a **specific monthly savings plan**. This restricts buying power in daily life. Consumption is thus limited, which is good for you – in the long term.

1. and 2.:   The current interest rate from the central banks for liquid money are down to or near zero – and this includes savings interest, which is close to zero too.
Insight: Money is melting like a glacier in bright sunlight due to inflation.
Inflation itself is needed to lubricate the economy – we spend money when its value deteriorates, but we would save it if the value was going to increase over night. Inflation is a driver for the markets – spend it before it's inflated.
This should be **emergency money** and should include only a small part of your funds. But **cash is king** if buying power is a matter of fact.

3.:   Life insurance companies are commercially-oriented companies doing business with calculated probabilities. To understand this, one must assume that this service is not for free, it costs money – your money. It is a kind of **tractor**, reliable but needing some of your money for fuel. Consider what would happen if you were short of money over the longer duration of 20 or 30 years and could not fulfill the payment. They're not too flexible.

4.:   An old friend of mine is in the real estate business in Vienna with his own construction team. He has made good money there. BUT, never forget the credits lines he had to draw from banking institutes to finance these projects. One must "have the balls" to take this big risk because a loss in a project would possibly leave him with losses and debts which the banks would call in, if necessary, by force. This can get dirty. This is too heavy for me and would've kept me awake at night ☹

But I followed his advice on a smaller scale:
- I learned how auctions work (dry run)
- I planned (place, area, my money, bank's money, what to invest and modernize and how to use the site later after renovation)
- I attended an auction and got what I bid on

- I organized the renovation, started the communication with the building management, organized electricity and gas, let the flat and included it in my tax declaration

Over the years the rental income pays back the credit line and increases my value.

But money in this fund is "frozen" and taking it out requires a "defrost" via a sale. To bet everything you have on something like this would completely immobilize you. **Real estate should only make up part of your funds.**

Saving studies in Austria (good old Europe) confirm the old pattern structure.

No Risk, No Fun: New Patterns

This brings us, inevitably, to the stock exchange. And so, the trouble begins!

- Which country or currency?
- Which company?
- Portfolio split?
- What about:
    - sell in May and come back in September?
    - don't touch a falling knife!
- Shares/bonds/funds/options?
- What about political impact?
- What is a stop-loss order?
- Interferences between interests and shares?
- Old business companies or new business companies?

Rethink the question when Morpheus in Matrix asks Neo to choose between:

- Blue pills   everything so far is known, nothing is new, comfort zone
- Red pills   awakening, risk and a lot of trouble and work and a bunch of learning stuff, no comfort zone, provided you are from good old Europe

Here, at the latest, you can choose the blue pill and return to your familiar environment!

Dow Jones

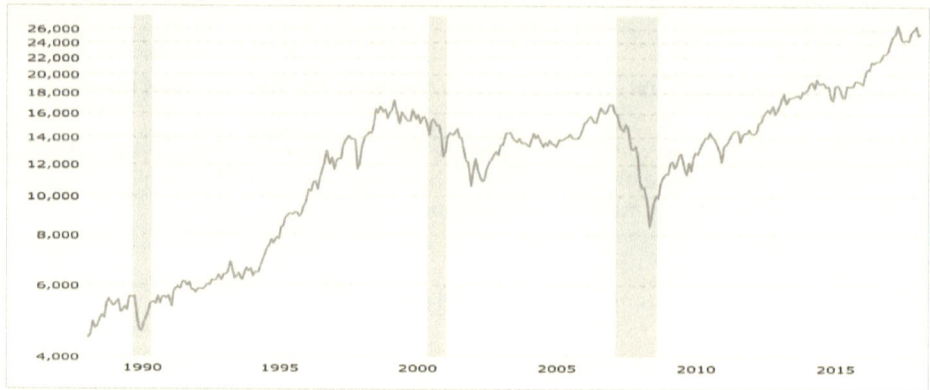

I'm fully with my daughter on this: <u>don't invest in something you don't understand.</u>
Everyone should stick to this and inform themselves prior to any new engagement.

Honestly, do you think that starting on this chart at approximately 5000 in 1990 and increasing the amount by fivefold in 2018 would have been possible when lending money to the bank? Never, ever!

Some insight from a starter:

+ Look at **disruptive companies** and give them a greater share of your portfolio than good old businesses.
+ **Copy the patterns of professional brokers**, e.g. *www.dirk-mueller-fonds.de*
  Be aware that the latter fund is more ark than speedboat.
+ Invest more in **bigger companies** than in smaller. Why? They can afford experts which are necessary for running businesses in a complex world. The smaller companies struggle more and fail more easily.
+ When investing for the **long term**, don't hop-on/hop-off, treat it like a bank account and consider the following:
  o Shares can be sold faster
  o Investment funds are to be sold in the long term or medium term based on their price construction (extra charge at the beginning)
  o Options grant some leverage – good or bad
+ **10 stocks should be enough**, providing a good overview and spread of risk.
+ Take a close look at market indicators that show stress and cut the line when:
  o Interest rises
  o Big company losses, debts rising, problems in repayment of loans, bank bankruptcy
  o Shortage of money

In the long term, reengineering your own energy system to save on long-term energy costs is another strategy. And it's good for the carbon footprint.

If you find yourself not ready to push the direct button to the stock exchange, then find a **professional broker** to do it for you. Provided they are reliable, they'll give you a **risk profile covering low to high risks.** So ... it's finally up to you to let the button be pushed.

<u>My own flops and errors:</u>

Having too little invested in cash and therefore being unable to take advantage of a karmic positive situation, i.e. a payment of 2 to 3 years earlier retirement for cheap money because my standard procedure was:

- have low debts which should be repaid as early as possible rather than having cash on hand and a little more debt. This was <u>too short-minded.</u>

Believing in a so called "soul hunter" selling a product named "loss participation model" who promised tax reductions. The result was:

- absolute loss
- tax deduction was declined

<u>Not understanding the whole construction process</u> adequately and trusting a friend who also didn't grasp the it completely ☹

<u>Acting like a dealer in buying today and selling two days later</u>, because a president said this or that, resulting in a loss that showed a lack in my ability to act in the short term – not the right stuff for a long-term thinking and acting man like me!

The stock exchange has brought me more success than the lottery!

CO$_2$

Global warming is a brutal reminder that borders are no protection for bad winds and bad weather. Last October I had anchored a sailing boat on the island of Lipari and was facing a very heavy storm. Anchoring in front of the island when a storm blows inland isn't the smartest thing one could do. Anyway, we had chosen this. The skipper and crew went blue awaiting redemption from the heavy waves. I was very frightened!

BUT, the water was lukewarm, in October! Nothing freezes. Even as the storm washed us ashore, our last steps were in warm water … in October!

Yep, I know some politicians are still captivated (by whom?) and tell us what is going on, treating us like illiterates. I have an inner resistance to using the main road, that's why I'm suspicious of this puppet theater.

Burning the sun's energy that has been stored in coal and mineral oils for millions of years within the space of a century will change the equation. To understand that millions of years are burned in a century, for example, doesn't require the brain of Albert Einstein. Common sense is enough but is necessary. Dr Joachim Schellnhuber, former head of the Potsdam Institute for Climate Impact Research, notes that increases of average temperatures by 5 degrees will lead to a drastic change of the biosphere and the extinction of countless species. This process needed some 10,000 years between the Permian and Triassic geological periods. We will achieve something similar, only much faster. This is like heading towards a wall with our only action being to take the foot off the accelerator, rather than apply a full emergency brake! Scientific wording for this behavior is "cognitive dissonance" which implies an unwillingness to face the ugly truth. He likens the result of our carbon dioxide production with the impact of an asteroid on earth.

The wording "climate change" further inflates the real significance of the problem. "Climate catastrophe" more realistically **addresses the problem**. Our minds will judge it more seriously. It's basic psychology.

Since our prosperity is based on energy consumption, mostly fossil fuels, what are our options?

I see two paths: my choice and our choice

My Choice:

1. **Isolate my house** or flat as much as possible or require the landlord to do so. Better isolation compensates for, to some extent, the need for air conditioning which requires a lot of energy. Use **solar panels** and use electricity for heating up warm water, laundry and dishwashing. Change your machines to lower consumption. I work a lot with timers to run machines during the day. My partner isn't always happy when I say: "Honey, let's do the laundry now, the sun is shining!"

2. Even constructing a **cistern** is helpful, providing water for toilet flushing, laundry and the backyard. In a very hot summer, it could be a saving grace to have stored water for the garden and for preventing the outbreak of fires. A capacity of 6 to 8 m^3 is enough to reduce flooding issues for the community in heavy storm conditions too!

3. Think global and buy local. Also buy seasonal goods. This results in:

a.

Meat

meat (a CO_2 trigger).

More vegetables than

No Meat

A small story about the total meat balance on our planet: Humans use up to 30%, livestock takes 67% and the rest (3%) is for our wildlife. Remember the vegetarian gorilla who is far stronger than any man without meat as protein source.

b. This is another puppet story – carnivores. When I was a teenager, the car safety belt was invented and everyone, including me, responded similarly: How do you get out of a car in an accident when fixed with a belt? No, this wouldn't work, and other stupid comments, as seen from my present knowledge point of view, followed. By the way, how should someone crawl out of a wrecked car when he himself is wrecked too. I finally took to the safety belt, but it was a long way to convince my grandfather who thought he was as strong as Superman. Withstanding gale forces from a sudden emergency break situation. My little calculation resulted in a ton to be deadlifted by two arms. Then he gave in. Hu.

It seems to be the same brain barrier with the meat/no meat button as the security belt.

Some more Greta's are needed to open new doors!

c. **Local and seasonal food rather** than exotic food reduces your carbon footprint.

d. **Organic vegetables** are healthier and use less protection mechanisms on the plants, meaning better energy efficiency.

My brother and his sons decided to run my father's farm as an organic farm – less artificial fertilizer, almost no insect and fungus protection. They get my blessing for this move!

4. Transport: I have an efficient car, of course, but do not use shared transport. In town, I bike for my daily need and use my backpack.

5. Use a bike for ride to the office. Instead of the car.

6. Avoid flying and use the night train instead.

7. Reduce consumption => reduce waste => reduction of energy consumption.

Our Choice

The greater community and our governments are responsible for correctly guiding people. This should include:

⇨ Higher taxation of non-renewable energy sources which means CO_2 taxes! According to a smart thinker, this must be started and constantly applied to change the human thinking pattern.
If it's done, it would be revolutionary. Chaos, as with the yellow vests protests in France, is most likely, not good.

In German the word for taxes is "Steuern" which is literally translated into "guiding". This means that guidance under the governmental umbrella is needed to steer the masses towards a better future.

⇨ Most important is a taxation on flight petrol.
⇨ Lower taxation or even subsidies for using renewable energy sources.
⇨ Coordinate this in a greater worldwide context.
⇨ Support the expansion of green energy resources.
⇨ Support the planting of tree belts around the world to reduce CO_2.

Mother Earth doesn't need mankind. Mankind needs Mother Earth.

DOWNLOADS

On www.fraanz.com you'll find some more hints and probably helpers.

DISCIPLINE

As I have already said:

1. My life is short. I am 58 this year and could expect 70 or 80 years in total.
    Then: game over. Time passes by like a quick river. Consequently, time is precious.

    Don't spoil this life with garbage, Samsara, consumption, constantly experiencing social media ... dear Franz!

2. I have learned a lot in my life (see the prior chapters)

To mix 1 and 2, DISCIPLINE is required!

Otherwise, the days are lost in distraction. Like an unguided missile. Whoosh, and one fire is wasted.

So, start with the end: a **life plan!**

Follow Arnolds Schwarzenegger's advice: **AIM high with your visions**. Your subconscious mind will find the practical milestones later, but if you don't aim high, you end low. Or, at least, average. Everyone must make their own decisions on how to deal with this unique LIFE. One is happy in his garden, the next one likes to save the world from air pollution or travelling around the globe. There is no single answer for everyone.

Find the goals that are important for you. My list:

- Be slim
- Flexibility of the body
- Cash on hand
- Create your own idea – like I have with this book
- Create the non-profit organization you always wanted to establish since you were a kid
- Fulfill your parent's deepest wishes, for e.g. by traveling at least once to Rome ...
- Bring quarrelling family members, partners and friends together
- Forgive your worst enemy for what they have done to you
- Build bridges and discover that, in the end, 1 + 1 is more than 2 when people get connected
- Learn the foreign language you always wanted to know
- Increase your endurance from potato hero to hobby athlete hero – it is possible

Digest these tasks faithfully and you'll realize that a lot must be done to bring the power of the brain to the road!

Nothing is for free, all must fully impact both brain and mood! This is not a shortcut, this needs FULL concentration! Find the right direction for you.

Avoid compromises. **Rather make a digital decision: 1 or 0.** Clear?
My fault was always doing something at 70% or even 40%, mixing too many things together and avoiding a clear direction, not accomplishing goals in a crystal-clear way!

Be a tough boss to yourself, but be softer on your disciples (kids, colleagues, etc.). This doesn't mean giving away principles for free, but rather shine by example. This way, your example can be seen and is practical.

Remember: **An ounce of practice is better** than tons of theory.
Therefore, the title of this book is "DO IT"

▲
▬ Avoid the naysayers: Again, advice from Arnold Schwarzenegger. If you are looking for the right company in life, you'll avoid the stoppers, the breakers, the limiters who'd never allow another to exceed the average. I call them the averagers. Anxious types crowd around the average, because this gives them a kind of team spirit for avoiding new ways. They prefer the known truth and don't expand their horizons. Hell, I know that 10 steps in entrepreneur mode into new areas includes 9 wrong steps or steps that don't fit. But not taking the crucial step would have resulted in not inventing the wheel or the moon rocket and not discovering America! THIS would have been the wrong turn. It is like freezing the present because this is the known. Or another crazy method is to avoid the next innovation step because in some years everything will be much newer and it's better to wait for that => never.

▲
▬ **A trick to avoid too much alcohol: 1 glass of water – then 1 glass of wine**
I often found myself in the evening thinking that I needed a glass of wine to come down, to relax. I have found that some easy breathing exercises or some yoga exercises have the same effect with no negative impact on health and power-levels. It was/is like turning a switch from alcohol to no alcohol. It's mostly a brain-setting which is stuck on old, and bad in this case, habits. This decision allowed me to write this book alongside my daily duties.

If you can climb a 2,000 m peak, **set the goal higher** – to 3,000 or 4,000 m!

If I'm able to complete a bike marathon of 85 km with 1 km up and down in three and a half hours, I set my goal to do it within 3 hours, or I must do a 120 km bike marathon!

The "entrance-fee" is simple: **10 kg less** ☺   No excuses.

RECAP

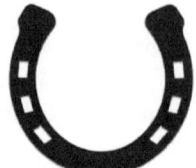

 Simplify your life

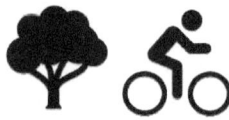 Consult Dr. Nature and Exercise (body & mind & soul)

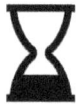 Slow gentle breathing breathes away problems and tension

16 / 8 The eating window is open for 8 hours – with lots of vegetables

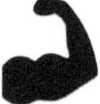 Trust in yourself

 Skip distractions

 **+ live your great visions and dreams**

+ DO IT